# *Fundamental Aspects of Long-Term Conditions*

 library

# Fundamental Aspects of Long-Term Conditions

A Guide for Students of Nursing and Health

*Edited by Helen McVeigh*

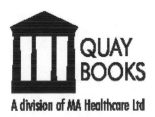

QUAY
BOOKS

A division of MA Healthcare Ltd

Quay Books Division, MA Healthcare Ltd, St Jude's Church, Dulwich Road, London
SE24 0PB

British Library Cataloguing-in-Publication Data
A catalogue record is available for this book

ISBN-10: 1 85642 392 1
ISBN-13: 978 1 85642 392 2

Printed by CLE, St Ives, Cambridgeshire

# Contents

Contents

# Contributors

**Jasmin Amoroso** MA, B. Ed (Hons) Practice Educator, Specialist Practitioner DN, RN
Senior Lecturer in Nursing, De Montfort University, Leicester

**Gill Ayling**
Full time carer

**Jacqui Day** MA, PG Dip Healthcare Education, RM, BA (Hons)
Senior Lecturer in Mental Health Nursing, De Montfort University, Leicester.
Jacqui is the academic lead for mental health within the university

**Ron Eldridge** MA, RGN, RMN, NDN Cert
Independent Nurse Prescriber and Community Matron, Leicester City Community Health Service

**Karen Ford** MSc, BSc(Hons), RHV, RGN
Senior Lecturer in Primary Care and Non-Medical Prescribing Lead,
De Montfort University, Leicester

**Chris Knifton** SBStJ, MSc, MA, LLB(Hons), BSc(Hons), FAETC, RNLD,
Dip SW, Dip AROM, Dip Counselling and Psychotherapy, Dementia Care Mapper (Adv)
Senior Lecturer in Nursing, De Montfort University, Leicester

**Deborah Lewis** MSc, RGN, DN Cert
Senior Lecturer in Cancer and Palliative Care, Birmingham City University
Faculty of Health, Edgbaston, Birmingham

**Jean Martey** RN, Independent Prescriber, City Guilds 7303
Parkinson's Disease Nurse Specialist; Secretary to the National Parkinson's Disease Nurse Association

**Helen McVeigh** MA Learning and Teaching, BSc (Hons) Community Health Nursing, RNT, RGN
Senior Lecturer in Primary Care, De Montfort University, Leicester

**Teresa Pratt** RNMH, Dip He Mental Health, BSc Specialist Nursing Practice (Mental Health), C & G Further and Adult Education Teachers' Certificate
Community Mental Health Nurse, Leicestershire Partnership Trust

**Paul Rigby** MA. BA (Hons). RMN. Dip Ad Ed. Dip Nurs. Dip Health Care Practice (THORN). Senior Lecturer
Senior Lecturer in Mental Health Nursing, De Montfort University, Leicester; Community Mental Health Team, Leicestershire Partnership NHS Trust

**Tony Robinson**
Person with Parkinson's

**Ruth Rojahn** MA Learning and Teaching, BA Nursing Practice, PG Dip (Educ), RGN, DN Cert, CPT (DN)
Senior Lecturer in Primary Care, De Montfort University, Leicester

**Janice Strefford** BSc (Hons) Community Health Nursing, RN
Practice Nurse

**Dr Ira Unell** PhD
Senior Lecturer in Substance Misuse and Course Director for the MSc in Drug and Alcohol Treatment at Leicester University Medical School

**Cheryl Utecht** MA, BA(Hons), RGN, ONC, DN(Cert)
Principal Lecturer at De Montfort University, Leicester

# Acknowledgements

I would like to express my appreciation to all those who supported me in this venture. To colleagues, practitioners and individuals who freely gave their time and agreed to contribute.

To John for his encouragement and support.

To Ruth for listening and proof reading.

To Gary for his patience and support.

*Helen McVeigh*
January 2010

# Foreword

Long-term conditions is an extremely important addition to the Fundamental Aspects series. The implication of increasing life expectancy is that many people now live with what have been termed 'long-term conditions'. Most people over the age of 50 years have some form of long-term health problem. For most, this is a relatively minor and easily treatable condition, such as raised blood pressure, some joint pain, eyesight deterioration, or mild diabetes, while for others the condition may be more serious.

Possibly one of the most distinguishing features of any long-term condition is the effect it has on the lifestyle not only of the person with the condition, but their family, friends and colleagues. This is brought out with considerable force in the chapters written by 'patients' and 'carers'. As nurses, so often we only see the immediate medical problem the patient is presenting with, and while that is important in terms of assessment and management, it must not be seen in isolation from the holistic picture, which so often, only the patient is aware of—hence the concept of the 'expert patient'.

In editing this book, Helen McVeigh has brought together a number of clinical specialists, university lecturers, patients with long-term conditions and carers. As you read through individual chapters and then the complete book, you will begin to appreciate not only the medical implications of long-term conditions, but in addition you will gain an insight to what it feels like to be labelled in this way. If you can have some empathy into that experience, then you will be a far more understanding nurse.

John Fowler
*Phd MA BA DipN Cert.Ed. RGN RMN RCNT RNT*
*Principal Lecturer in Nursing*
*De Montfort University*
*Series Editor*
*Fundamental Aspects of Nursing*

# Introduction

Providing support and care for individuals with a long-term condition is an essential feature of modern health care. Over 15 million people in England currently have a long-term condition, and it is predicted that these numbers will continue to rise (Department of Health [DH], 2008). The impact of long-term conditions will affect every one of us in some way. For many of us this may be first hand as a sufferer, for others it will be in providing care or support to a partner, family member or friend.

The DH defines long-term conditions as 'those that cannot at present be cured but can be controlled by medication or other therapies' (DH, 2007). Living with a chronic illness offers no rosy end-point; unlike acute illness, where full recovery is expected, there is no return to normal health. The length, progress and severity of the illness will mean that the individual has to come to terms with living with their condition. For the individual this will often necessitate lifestyle changes and modifying expectations for the future.

As nurses, our understanding of how a long-term condition influences an individual is often guided by our medical and physical knowledge of disease processes. We need to remember that living with a chronic illness will impact on all aspects of life. There will be significant psychological, social and emotional costs of living with a long-term condition. A holistic nursing perspective acknowledges that practice should be underpinned with a comprehensive understanding of all factors that impact on the quality of life for an individual; physiological, psychological, social, spiritual and environmental. We also need to understand and acknowledge the experiential experiences of the individuals we care for. In addition, nursing practice needs to evolve in response to the changing expectations of individuals, society and healthcare provision. Our success in providing effective and long-lasting quality interventions may well be reliant on successfully balancing our understanding of all these aspects of care.

This book aims to raise your awareness of long-term conditions, their management and the implications of living with chronic illness. The book takes a patient-centred, holistic approach, which aims to help you understand that an individual's response to having a long-term condition is both complex and unique to them. The focus throughout explores long-term conditions in relation to the adult patient. Although some long-term conditions may begin in childhood, the concept of disease management in childhood and the implications this raises is considered to be a separate topic.

Chapter 1 introduces the subject and places long-term conditions in context, and looks at the impact current policy has on healthcare provision. It explores the notion of chronic illness and identifies a framework for management which introduces the concepts of self-care and the expert patient. The themes raised in this chapter are echoed in the approach and structure of subsequent chapters.

The following chapters focus on specific conditions taking a proactive approach that considers management, the role of relevant services, coping strategies, quality of life and self-management. While chapters have focused on individual conditions, it is important to be aware that many individuals may have more than one condition, or indeed complex comorbidities. It is also important to recognize that many conditions will shorten life expectancy and chapter 14 considers the topic of palliative care and end-of-life decisions. The issue of lifestyle choice and the influence this has on both the development of and progress of long-term conditions is of particular relevance. Chapters 12 and 13 explore the issues of obesity and alcohol use, while smoking is discussed within Chapter 5 in relation to chronic obstructive pulmonary disease (COPD).

Management is not just the remit of health care, as living with a long-term condition affects all aspects of a persons' life; home, work, relationships, environment, spirituality, and psychological wellbeing. The 'real life' impact of living with a long-term condition is considered in Chapter 8, which highlights the personal reflection of a patient. Coping with chronic illness impacts on the quality of life of not only the individual concerned and Chapter 9 emphasizes the personal reflection of a carer. A coordinated approach involving the patient, carers, primary care, secondary care, and social care provision is fundamental to effective management strategies and the provision of high quality care that meets the needs of both the individual and communities. Chapter 15 explores the concept of multi-professional collaboration and identifies the myriad of services that are available to support individuals in managing their conditions, while Chapter 16 considers the future and the use of technology in managing and supporting health care.

# Using this book

The chapters of this book have been designed with a structured approach. Chapters are introduced with a list of suggested learning outcomes. Each chapter highlights the epidemiology and demography of specific conditions and draws attention to relevant policy supporting health care. A needs-led focus on the patient is used, including physical, social, psychological, spiritual, cultural, and environmental issues. Many of the contributors have used case history examples and scenarios to illustrate aspects of need and the issues discussed. Within each chapter, you will find questions related to content and points for reflection.

This book sets a challenge to student nurses and those embarking on their nursing career pathway, that supporting patients with long-term conditions is the responsibility of all nurses. An individualized, person-centred approach is fundamental to care provision. This book should make you think about how you can make a difference in the lives of those managing with a long-term condition. It should enable you to take a holistic perspective in the care, management and support of these patients.

'When you leave the clinic you still have a long term condition, when the visiting nurse leaves your home you still have a long term condition. In the middle of the night you fight the pain alone. At the weekend you manage without your home help. Living with a long term condition is a great deal more than medical or professional assistance.'

Department of Health (2005:2).

# References

DH (2005) *Supporting people with long term conditions. An NHS and social care model to support local innovation and integration.* DH, London. ref: 4230

DH (2007) Long-term conditions: Background. http://tinyurl.com/kw6n3v (accessed 15 December 2009)

DH (2008) *Raising the profile of long term conditions: A compendium of information.* DH, London. ref: 8734

# Long-term conditions in context

*Helen McVeigh*

The management of long-term conditions is a great challenge for the health services. This chapter places long-term conditions in context by exploring the factors influencing the effective management of chronic disease, and identifying the policies that underpin the drive to provide appropriate services to meet this need. It examines the role of practitioners in meeting this agenda and highlights some of the challenges and problems that may arise.

Reading this chapter and reflecting on your own experiences should enable you to achieve the following learning outcomes:

- An understanding of how long term conditions can be effectively managed and the implications for healthcare provision
- A raised awareness of the policies and strategies underpinning the long term conditions agenda
- Identify the roles and scope of practice of health professionals in managing long-term conditions
- An insight into the concept of self-management.

## Background

Since its inception in 1948, the NHS has aimed to provide a service that offers high quality health care based on a core principle to meet the needs of everyone, regardless of the ability to pay. In recent years, the Government has recognized that the biggest challenge to healthcare provision lies in the effective management of long-term conditions. Approximately 15.4 million people in England are living with a long-term condition—this figure equates to approximately 60% of the adult population (Office for National Statistics [ONS], 2006). The majority of these individuals are likely to be elderly. Estimates suggest that three quarters of those over 75 years will suffer from chronic illness and half of those will have more than one condition (Department of Health [DH], 2005a). There is also inequity in the distribution of chronic disease as incidence is frequently higher in disadvantaged communities (DH, 2008a).

It is important to consider the root causes of the high burden of chronic disease. Twentieth century advancements have made fundamental changes to the demographic make-up of our population. The Western world has seen increasing life expectancy, falling birth rates in developed countries and an increasing older population, in part a result of the post-war 'baby boom' generation reaching retirement age. Forecasts indicate that the level of chronic disease is set to increase, with the percentage of those over 65 years of age living with a long-term condition likely to double by 2030 (World Health Organization [WHO], 2005). This problem is not just confined to the Western world. Globally, 60% of all deaths can be attributed to chronic disease (WHO, 2005). Projections for 2030 indicate that three out of the four leading causes of global mortality will be a result of chronic disease, notably ischaemic heart disease, cerebrovascular disease (stroke), and chronic obstructive pulmonary disease (COPD) (WHO, 2007).

---

### Reflection

* Consider why there has been an increase in life expectancy
* What health and social factors may have influenced this?

---

The past century has seen huge changes in our living and working environments, with better working conditions, improvements in housing and sanitation, and a raised awareness of public health. In 1901, life expectancy was only 48.5 years for men and 52.4 years for women, and mortality rates indicate that infectious disease was the most common cause of death, with 25% attributable to respiratory infectious disease (Griffiths and Brock, 2003; ONS, 2008a). Premature death was also a significant factor, with infant mortality accounting for 25% of all deaths (Griffiths and Brock, 2003). Early 20th century advances saw the introduction of new medicines, the development of antibiotics, the development of insulin, and the implementation of mass immunization and vaccination programmes. Increasing wealth and accessibility to a variety of foods has influenced diet and nutrition.

Furthermore, since the introduction of the NHS in 1948, there have been great advances in clinical science and significant technologies that enable us

| Table 1.1 The impact of ageing and disease on life expectancy | | |
| --- | --- | --- |
| | **Healthy (years)** | **Disability-free (years)** |
| *At birth* | | |
| Males | 67.9 | 62.3 |
| Females | 70.3 | 63.9 |
| *By age 65 years* | | |
| Males | 12.5 | 9.9 |
| Females | 14.5 | 10.7 |
| Adapted from: Office for National Statistics (2008b) Crown Copyright source: UK Statistics Authority, www.statistics.gov.uk | | |

to live for longer. Surgery has become increasingly sophisticated, medicines and treatments have been developed to control and limit the progression of disease, computerized technology has revolutionized communication, while screening and immunization programmes help to prevent or identify disease earlier. Current life expectancy in the UK is 76.9 years for men and 81.3 years for women (ONS, 2008b). The impact of ageing and living with chronic disease can be seen if we look at these figures in relation to healthy life expectancy and disability-free life (*Table 1.1*).

As well as an increased life expectancy, personal health expectations have been raised—we all want the opportunity to live high-quality, healthy lives, free from illness and disability. Our aspirations for the future in terms of our own health may be to live longer, but also to live better; in other words, we expect a higher quality of health. However, not all advances have led to a healthier, longer life, as some of the lifestyle choices we make have negatively impacted on the burden of chronic disease, placing increasingly high risk on the development of chronic conditions. Evidence shows that respiratory deaths are no longer high as a result of infectious disease, but risk factors such as smoking have elevated their incidence and tobacco-related death is likely to be responsible for around 10% of deaths globally by 2015 (WHO, 2007). Nutritional excesses and the availability of cheaper products high in fat have led to rising levels of obesity, accounting for at least one death in every 13 within the EU (Banegas et al, 2003).

The effective management of long-term conditions is highlighted as a key priority of the DH. People with a long-term condition are disproportionate users of the NHS (Wilson et al, 2005). Figures indicate that:

- 2% of patients with long-term conditions account for around 30% of unplanned hospital admissions (DH, 2005b)
- 80% of GP consultations relate to long-term conditions (Scott, 2004)

- 5% of inpatients account for 49% of all inpatient bed days (DH, 2008a)
- 72% of all hospital bed days are for patients with a long-term condition (DH, 2008a)
- An estimated 50% of medication is not taken as prescribed (DH, 2005c).

Approximately 78% of healthcare spending in the UK can be linked with the management of long-term conditions. If we also consider projections for an increasing ageing population, it is likely that in the future this figure will rise (Fletcher, 2005; DH, 2008a). In fact, by 2020 the WHO predict that chronic disease will be the primary cause of disability and the most costly problem for health services, not only in the UK, but worldwide (WHO, 2002; 2005).

To meet these spiralling needs, the Government identified a framework aimed at improving care for those with long-term conditions (DH, 2004a; 2005b). The foundations for this policy direction were initiated within the *NHS Plan* (DH, 2000) and echoed in the *National Service Framework for Long-Term Conditions* (DH, 2005c), which highlighted the need to focus healthcare priorities towards effectively managing long-term conditions:

*'... to improve health outcomes for people with long-term conditions by offering a personal care plan for vulnerable people most at risk; and to reduce emergency bed days by 5% by 2008 through improved care in primary care and community settings.'*

*Department of Health (2005b: 3)*

Identified aims include ensuring communities have an effective approach to the care and management of long-term conditions, reducing the reliance on secondary care, strengthening primary care provision, and ensuring care is patient-led and personalized to individual requirements. This policy direction clearly shifts the responsibility for the effective management of long-term conditions into the primary care arena. Although key aims are the improvement of health, underlying aims are focused on reducing the financial burden of avoidable healthcare use and particularly within secondary care (Dixon et al, 2004; Hunter, 2005). *Our Health, Our Care, Our Say* (DH, 2006) and *Choosing Health* (DH, 2004b) make it clear that better preventive and earlier intervention strategies are integral to improved health and wellbeing. In addition, increasing control and personal choice for individuals over their healthcare needs, and improving access to services and tackling health inequalities are highlighted as central to providing effective services. *Our Vision for Primary and Community Care* (DH, 2008b) indicates that by 2010 all 15.4 million people with a long-term condition should have a personalized care plan to support their needs. Lord Darzi (DH, 2008c) notes that 'giving patients more control over their care including the information

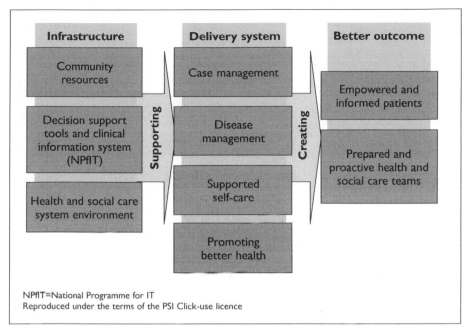

| Infrastructure | Delivery system | Better outcome |

Community resources

Case management

Empowered and informed patients

Decision support tools and clinical information system (NPfIT)

Supporting

Disease management

Creating

Prepared and proactive health and social care teams

Supported self-care

Health and social care system environment

Promoting better health

NPfIT=National Programme for IT
Reproduced under the terms of the PSI Click-use licence

*Figure 1.1. The NHS and social care long-term conditions model (From: DH, 2005b)*

to make healthy choices ... will reduce their chances of poor health and dependency on the NHS' (DH, 2008c: 37). Overall, policy direction is underpinned by an approach that reflects aspirations for healthier futures.

The framework for managing long-term conditions, the 'NHS and social care model' (DH, 2005b), identifies an infrastructure using a range of resources: the health and social care environment, local community resources, decision support tools, and clinical information systems (*Figure 1.1*). Management is met through a variety of levels of care:

- Case management
- Disease management
- Supported self-care
- Promoting better health.

The model aspires to better prepared and proactive health and social care teams, and strives for better informed and empowered patients. Overall aims focus on the following principles (DH, 2005b; 2008a):

- Earlier detection of chronic disease
- Good control to minimize the effects and reduce complications from chronic disease processes

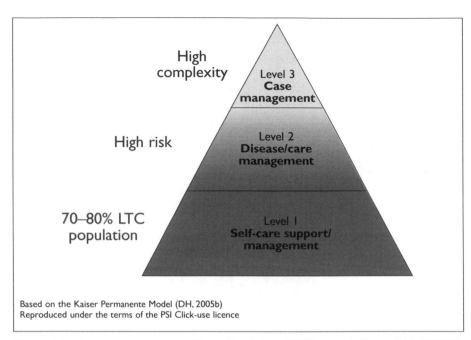

*Figure 1.2. Delivery system Long-Term Conditions (LTC) model (From: DH, 2005b)*

- Provide effective medicines management
- Reduce the number of crises for patients
- Promotion of independence and the empowerment of patients
- Prolong and extend the quality of life for those with a long-term condition.

The delivery system examines the profile and needs of patients with long-term conditions within the UK. The results can be viewed as a triangle with the bulk of patients living with a long-term condition capable of self-management and situated at the bottom tier of the triangle, while the 3–5% of those with the most complex needs occupy the top tier (*Figure 1.2*).

Analysis of the composition of the needs of these individuals indicates that support and/or intervention may be required on three levels (DH, 2005b):

- Level 1: approximately 70–80% of those with long-term conditions, those requiring more support to self-manage
- Level 2: high-risk patients who need active management and ongoing monitoring or review
- Level 3: approximately 3–5% of those with complex, often multiple conditions who require a case management approach.

The overall objective is to target health intervention according to level and type of need. Those individuals identified as the highest risk are inevitably the most frequent users of NHS resources and may require more intensive support.

## What is a long-term condition?

If we are examining long-term conditions, it is useful to define what we mean by chronic illness. In the simplest terms, it is illness that cannot be cured or as put in the words of one patient, 'something that does not get better, it is always there'. As such, managing subsequent health care moves away from traditional expectations as a health professional, to improve health or make someone better. We need to recognize that managing long-term conditions is a complex and life-long process for which the health professional may provide greater or lesser input at any one time. Although we acknowledge that chronic disease and illness may mean there is no cure, the great majority of people diagnosed with a chronic condition only seek to proactively manage their illness when they feel unwell. Although some chronic disease is characterized by ever-present symptoms, for others (e.g. diabetes, coronary heart disease) the asymptomatic element may lead patients to deny the existence and increases the potential for making inappropriate health/lifestyle choices. For many patients with a long-term condition, what is important is to know the difference between feeling well and being well.

Consider the chronic asthma sufferer who feels well and is able to take part in all the work and leisure activities he/she would like to, apart from occasional breathlessness on exertion. This person may only access healthcare support at times of ill-health (e.g. a chest infection following influenza), which has caused an exacerbation in his/her symptoms. Patients require assistance to maintain their health status even if they are fully aware of their illness and the impact this has on them. The challenge to the health professional lies in identifying the level of support required and being able to access those individuals to offer timely advice or intervention. Consider again the asthmatic person whose medication includes both preventive treatment (e.g. Seretide, beclametasone) and that giving instant relief (e.g. salbutamol); at the notion of feeling well, he/she has stopped taking his/her preventive medicine a number of weeks/months before the acute episode of a chest infection. Patients often require ongoing support to understand their condition and the implications of the choices they make. In making their choices, it is important they can make an informed decision or, as Gawande (2007) notes, that they know which odds they are playing. The challenge is to find the balance between providing health advice and support in ways which are acceptable and understandable, and to acknowledge that decisions are often made in the context of not only the knowledge of their disease, but beliefs, values, responsibilities, and personal choice.

Many patients will have more than one condition, particularly when examining the profile of those with advancing age. In some cases one condition may lead to the development of another. For example, poorly-controlled diabetes may lead to renal failure. Although there are a myriad of conditions that come under the umbrella of a 'long-term condition', the main focus of service provision is targeted at those conditions that are either more prevalent and/or impact highly in terms of financial burden to the NHS. Coronary heart disease accounts for 1 in 5 deaths in men and 1 in 6 in women (ONS, 2008b); nearly 7 million people in the UK are hypertensive (Quality and Outcomes Framework [QOF], 2006/07); heart failure affects around 707 000 (Allender et al, 2008); there are 2.5 million diabetics in the UK, with projections that this will rise to 3 million by 2012 (Diabetes UK, 2009); there are 766 000 COPD sufferers who are the most expensive users of NHS budget (British Thoracic Society, 2006); and there are around 8.5 million people in the UK with arthritis (Arthritis Research Campaign [ARC], 2009). Although it is paramount that these highly visible conditions are effectively targeted, it is equally important that health provision considers the needs of all those with a long-term condition.

## Case management

The 3–5% of high-risk patients identified as those with more complex needs require intensive support using a case management approach. Case management describes a proactive approach to care delivery, which will identify those individuals with a long-term condition who are most at risk and facilitates the management of care in partnership with the individual and their carers (NHS National Workforce Projects, 2006). The case manager coordinates the patient's journey through health and social care services using a holistic approach that encompasses assessment, planning and the delivery of individualized care. Scott (2004) suggests this role of care coordinator can be likened to that of a 'search engine in human form', enabling patients to effectively negotiate their path through the NHS. Case management principles highlighted in the Government's long-term condition agenda indicate that the community matron would act as the case manager. The fundamental aims of this role are to improve quality of life and ensure that a patient's condition remains stable (DH, 2005a). Factors such as being adaptable to the needs of local communities, and the role of educating other health professionals and local agencies in the proactive management of long-term conditions are also significant (Billingham, 2005).

The role and scope of the community matron is a significant evolutionary step for primary care nursing. Although there may be local variations in the interpretation of the role across the country, a community matron is an experienced and skilled nurse who will provide advanced nursing care combined with case management in order to improve quality of life, maintain wellbeing and manage acute exacerbations of those with complex needs in chronic disease (DH, 2005a). Working as a high-level practitioner with complex care packages requires additional competency and a wide range of skills (*Table 1.2*). To function effectively, these should include (DH, 2005d):

- Diagnostic and assessment skills
- Aetiology and treatment options
- Skills in change management
- The role of primary care in managing acute sector demand
- Case management principles
- Medicines management and experience in nurse prescribing.

The community matron will typically have a small caseload of patients (approximately 50) who require intensive support (DH, 2005a). An important element in meeting the needs of these patients is identifying the target population. A range of methodology to identify those at risk is used and predictive risk tools, such as the Patients at Risk of Re-hospitalisation (PARR) tool (The King's Fund, 2005), which identifies those with significant risk factors and those who have concurrent, frequent or increased risk of hospital admission, are used. In addition, the Combined Predictive Model identifies those at risk who have never had an admission (The King's Fund, 2006). There are flaws in any system that predicts levels of risk related to readmission. Many factors can influence this (Roland et al, 2005), and the community matron may use additional strategies including analysis of general practice computer systems, local knowledge, and liaison with other agencies to identify patient caseload.

Once identified, the community matron's role includes:

- Implementing an individualized package of care that focuses on individual assessment and care planning
- Regular and proactive monitoring
- Identified interventions

## Table 1.2 Core competencies for case management

| Domain | Additional competencies |
| --- | --- |
| Advanced clinical nursing practice | Medical history-taking<br>Advanced clinical nurse practitioner<br>Initiate and interpret diagnostic tests<br>Critical reasoning<br>Diagnose<br>Decision-making<br>Independent prescriber |
| Leading complex care coordination | Proactively coordinate and organize complex care packages<br>Support personalized care plan delivery<br>Monitor care provided |
| Proactively manage long-term conditions | Facilitate informed decision-making<br>Risk management |
| Managing cognitive impairment and mental wellbeing | Undertake basic assessment of mental health<br>Identify and assess deteriorating cognitive functioning<br>Recognize deterioration in mental wellbeing |
| Supporting self-care, self-management and enabling independence | Enable and promote independence |
| Professional practice and leadership | Maintain continuing competent practice at advanced level |
| Identifying high-risk patients, promoting health and preventing ill-health | Identify high-intensity user caseload<br>Promote health-enhancing behaviour<br>Prevent further deterioration in indentified caseload |
| Managing care at the end of life | Working with individuals in planning for the future and making choices about end-of-life care |
| Interagency and partnership working | Leading and working across organizational and professional boundaries |

Adapted from: DH (2005d)

- Education of patients and their families/carers
- Coordinating service provision
- Liaison with other agencies
- Evaluation of patient outcomes.

The community matron role involves not only identifying those at risk, but responding to ongoing risks and identifying what these may be in the context of patient life choices. It may be that a patient will choose high-risk behaviour on balance against the benefits of other available choices. What is important is that these choices are informed. In other words, the matron can close the gap between knowledge and the choices made. The community matron also has a significant role in identifying patients' coping strategies. Techniques such as motivational interviewing can be useful to initiate and sustain change in lifestyle and behaviours (Masterson, 2007a; Furze et al, 2008). They require skills in acting as a patient advocate and may attend outpatient appointments with a patient, for example. The importance of developing a good rapport with the patient is essential as the community matron will frequently be the first link in a chain of support within complex primary health and social care provision, or the first point of contact for vulnerable individuals when conditions are unstable or at times of exacerbation. It is also important that the community matron is able to recognize when the levels of support and intervention can be reduced so that ongoing care and support can be delegated to and managed by other primary care services.

## Disease management

The role of community matron focuses on greatest need, typically within the top 5% of patients with a long-term condition (DH, 2005a). Nurses in primary care will have the responsibility to support those individuals who make up the majority of patients with a long-term condition. At level 2, there are a significant number of patients who are at high risk because their condition is unstable, or who are more likely to deteriorate without appropriate support and will therefore require specific disease management (DH, 2005b). The aim of care for this group of patients is to provide responsive, specialist services using multi-disciplinary teams and disease–specific care pathways (DH, 2005b). Identifying patients who require this level of support can be problematic, and information from the general practice computer system and QOF data can be used to identify those with a long-term condition. A significant number may already be known to members of the primary care team, or will have been identified for ongoing support by the community matron once they no longer need this level of care. Support for these individuals can come from district nursing teams through ongoing care packages, and within practice nursing by regular proactive review. The approach to care and ongoing management at this level needs to reflect holistic principles of care that are patient-centred and underpinned by a care-planning approach. Effective care planning can be seen as a 'dynamic route map guiding the process of care' (NHS Modernisation Agency, 2005). It can improve the continuity of care provision, aid the identification and management of risk factors, and facilitate supported self-care. It is clear that effective proactive management of individuals at this level may prevent them from becoming unwell enough to require more intensive care. It could be argued, therefore, that those with the most significant role in managing long-term conditions are those that meet patients at levels 1 and 2 (*Figure 1.2*).

Nurses are recognized as best placed to meet the needs of those with a long-term condition (Hunter, 2005). However, the management of long-term conditions is not just the remit of the community matron and community nursing teams. Nurses will come into contact with people with chronic illness within all walks of life — in occupational health, in residential and nursing homes, in prisons — and these individuals may also access secondary care, whether this is for an acute exacerbation of illness or for elective surgery not necessarily associated with the condition. The opportunities for health professionals to provide support and direction may need to be more opportunistic so that the principles of managing, supporting and initiating health promotion and preventive strategies become embedded in everyday health care, from all aspects and within all professional groups. All healthcare practitioners have a role to play, whether this is the healthcare assistant, the student nurse at the 'coal face', the staff nurse, or the director of nursing.

## Supported self-care

The majority of individuals with a long-term condition (70–80%) can be supported to develop the skills, knowledge and confidence to manage their condition. There is a need to move away from a traditional model of paternalistic health care where 'doctor knows best', which does not fit with the long-term conditions model, to proactive self-management within a framework of supportive health care. Issues such as individualized care and patient choice have become central to current healthcare provision. What would we include as self-care?

> *'Self care includes everything people undertake to; maintain their health, prevent illness, seek and adhere to treatment, manage symptoms and side effects, accomplish recovery and rehabilitation and manage the impact of long term illness and disability.'*
>
> *Alliance for Self Care Research (2008)*

Nursing has always sought to be a profession focused on holistic principles, which endeavours to consider all aspects of care provided. Management of chronic disease should extend beyond physiological–reactive responses to encompass social and personal needs and values. The patient with a long-term condition may require support which reflects all aspects of health and social care in order to meet their needs effectively. Although secondary care provision and specialist nurses have an important role to play in meeting these needs, it is of equal importance that ongoing care and management be incorporated into primary care provision. In reality, the individual with a long-term condition will spend most of his/her life living and working, and only accessing secondary care services to meet exacerbations of their condition or in emergency situations. It is important to remember that contact with primary care services may also be very limited. If we consider a diabetic patient, the typical length of contact time they will have with a health professional (assuming they are not acutely unwell) will be 3 hours per year. For the rest of the year he/she will be self-caring. Opportunities may exist to provide support and/or management, or simply identifying problems in every communication we have with a patient. Reflection on practice can enable us to identify where these opportunities lie. For example, consider the patient admitted for elective surgery who identifies a long-term condition in the process of admission, or the same patient who attends his/her local surgery for the removal of sutures. Should we be asking, 'Have I done any more than simply taking a patient history and/or removing the sutures?'

Supporting self-management is based on being able to develop a good relationship with the patient that also respects his/her personal values and belief systems. As health professionals, we need to be aware that effective management of a long-term condition will frequently require the individual to change his/her behaviour. Therefore, it is important to recognize that successful achievement of self-management may depend on a readiness, willingness and ability to change (Masterson, 2007a). This requires an understanding of how the concept of compliance *vs* concordance may influence the effectiveness of any advice and support given:

- Compliance: adherence to directions given by a health professional (Koch et al, 2004)
- Concordance: based on a partnership between patient and health professional. Focus is on shared decision-making that respects the beliefs, values and wishes of the patient (Brooker, 2006).

As nurses, our understanding and knowledge of the risk factors and how these will affect health outcomes in relation to chronic conditions may lead us to use a compliance-focused approach to health education and supportive advice. This may be an appropriate method for some individuals, for example older patients who may expect a more paternalistic style in which the nurse tells them what to do (Koch et al, 2004). However, a concordant approach reflects a true partnership between patient and nurse that respects the views of the individual, allowing him/her to make truly informed choices. This can empower the individual and allow him/her to retain control of his/her health. Long-term conditions are frequently influenced by lifestyle choices. The choices made in relation to health care are frequently made through a process of balancing the personal gains against the risk taken. Enabling patients to recognize and identify these risks, and make positive choices, can be key to the effective management of a chronic condition (Masterson, 2007a).

It could be argued that in order to ensure the health of those with a long-term condition, greater levels of monitoring and an increase in health service provision are required. Effective self-management can also be seen as cost-effective and as such, an important factor in efficient resource management. However, increasing the amount of proactive contact and appointments can have a negative effect. It may be seen as overly-intrusive on a persons' life, or as removing the ability for him/her to make his/her own life choices. In reality, by facilitating effective self-care we are mobilizing a workforce that is much greater than the health service can offer (Expert Patients Programme Community Interest Company [EPP CIC], 2007a; DH, 2009).

## Expert patient

It is recognized that individuals who have lived with their condition for a significant length of time may, by virtue of their experiences, be regarded as experts (DH, 2001). The expert patient concept recognizes that over time, patients are likely to develop expertise in managing their condition (DH, 2001). Although health professionals have the relevant medical knowledge, there may be a lack of understanding of how this impacts on the realities of everyday life. Recent surveys (DH, 2005e; 2006) indicated that 86% of respondents thought that professionals in their local GP practice should provide more support to help them take care of their own health, but 33% indicated that they thought the support for self-care should come from a peer. Self-care needs to be a real choice for patients. All too frequently the reality of managing a long-term condition will lead to long-term dependence. The benefits of effective self-care can be gauged in real terms. Statistics from the ONS (2008b) reported that improved self-care could have resulted in 10 000 less heart attacks, 5000 less deaths, and 1000 fewer operations, not to mention the additional benefits to patients in extended and improved quality of life.

The Expert Patients Programme was established by the DH (2001) and is now under the management of the EPP CIC, which was launched in April 2007. It is a not-for-profit organization underpinned by the values of social enterprise, i.e. any profit made is put back into the organization for the benefit of the organization. It delivers self-management and support courses, and supports other organizations in the delivery of self-management across a range of long-term conditions. It operates on the principle that an individual is an active manager in their own care and aims to help them minimize the symptoms and effects of living with a chronic illness (EPP CIC, 2007a).

*'The Expert Patients Programme will help to create a new generation of patients who are empowered to take action in partnership with the health professional caring for them, for example, to reduce pain, to improve the use of medication, and enhance their overall quality of life. Patients will receive support to help them take more control of their own health and treatment, to make more appropriate use of health and social services, and become more empowered.'*
*Expert Patient Programme Community Interest Company (2007b: vii)*

Self-care is about individuals taking responsibility for their own health and wellbeing. If people have a clearer understanding of their condition, they are more likely to take control and be proactively involved.

---

### Reflection

Think about a patient you have met with a long-term condition
- Consider all aspects of their condition from physiological, psychological, and social and environmental perspectives
- Consider what self-management abilities this patient may have
- What type of support would they need to become effective in the self-management of their condition?

## Collaborative working

It is not possible to meet the needs of individuals from within a single health or social care profession (Walsh et al, 2005). Delivering truly individualized care for patients with a long-term condition requires a multi-professional approach. To ensure the delivery of patient-centred care based on the principles of holism, the ability of health professionals to work together is paramount (Glen, 2004). However, this will require effective communication and collaborative skills (Hutt et al, 2004) to effectively integrate services across the whole of the health and social care network.

Nurses clearly have a key role to play in the management of long-term conditions, but this should not be in isolation or too narrowly focused. Case management and the community matron's role is based on a medically-focused model, which could overlook the skills and expertise of other professionals (Hunter, 2005). Chronic illness impacts on all aspects of life and this raises the question of whether the nurse has the relevant knowledge to support and advise on issues such as benefits, housing or education; issues which may be of particular relevance when viewed in conjunction with the evidence indicating that the highest incidence of long-term conditions is found in the most disadvantaged groups (e.g. unemployed, areas of social deprivation) (DH, 2008a). The community matron or primary care nurse may need exceptional skills in order to expertly coordinate and manage care provision that requires both a broad knowledge of different services, as well as an increasing need for specialization (Walsh et al, 2005). Nurses need to work alongside and with other professions, and consider how they can facilitate the inclusion of relevant social care skills to ensure effective care planning and case management.

Effective interprofessional collaboration presents a challenge to all. Breaking down barriers between health and social care and facilitation of cross-boundary working may not be an easy task. Without effective collaboration, support for those with a long-term condition can be hampered by fragmentation of care and duplication of assessment procedures. There may also be confusion and a lack of clarity of the role and responsibilities of those involved and an unnecessary waste of valuable resources, which will inevitably impact on the quality of care provided. Issues such as poor communication, lack of trust and confidence in other agencies, professional ideology, service hierarchies and differing value systems are recognized barriers to successful collaboration (Doyle, 2008; Jelphs and Dickinson, 2008; Miers and Pollard, 2009). Improving methods of communication, developing an understanding of the roles and responsibilities of different professions, and building effective teamwork skills can promote interprofessional collaboration (Masterson, 2007b;

Doyle, 2008; Miers and Pollard, 2009). It is important to remember that the quality of patient care may be positively influenced, not only by individual professionals' expertise, but also by the way professionals work with each other (Camsooksai, 2002).

*'The best care and support is delivered by professionals working together as part of teams to meet the needs of communities, groups and individuals.'*

*Department of Health (2008c: 5)*

## Conclusion

This chapter has explored the background to providing support for those with a long-term condition. The evidence shows that people with long-term conditions are intensive users of health and social care services, and that the size of the problem is set to increase given the ageing population and peoples' lifestyle choices (DH, 2008a). It is necessary for healthcare provision to target the management of chronic conditions in order to provide effective health care. The long-term conditions model (DH, 2005b) provides a framework for the delivery of health and social care provision in meeting this need. Management and care of those with a long-term condition is delivered according to the level and complexity of a patient's needs and focuses on case management, disease management and supported self-care. A patient-centred approach should be the over-arching philosophy. Negotiating care plans, providing support and recognizing when and how a patient may be able to self-care are fundamental to improving patient outcomes.

Although the community matron has a significant role to play in the management of those with the most complex needs, effective support and care for the majority of those with a chronic condition is firmly in the remit of all nurses working in primary care. The challenge to provide high quality and effective care and support for individuals with chronic conditions is multifaceted and also requires a coordinated approach from professionals across all areas of health and social care. Good teamwork, a partnership approach, and strategies to meet this are integral for interprofessional collaboration. It is essential that the nurse is aware of his/her role and responsibilities in supporting those individuals with a long-term condition within the scope of his/her professional practice.

*'Delivering improvements for people with long term conditions isn't just about treating illness, it's about delivering personalised, responsive, holistic care in the full context of how people want to live their lives.'*

*Department of Health (2008a: 5)*

Allender S, Peto V, Scarborough P, Kaur A, Rayner M (2008) Coronary Heart Disease Statistics 2008. http://tinyurl.com/da8o5t (accessed 8 December 2009)

Alliance for Self Care Research (2008) About Self-care. www.ascr.ac.uk/selfcare.htm (accessed 25 September 2009)

Arthritis Research Campaign (2009) UK Arthritis facts—at a glance. http://tinyurl.com/ycr2cll (accessed 25 September 2009)

Banegas JR, López-García E, Gutiérrez-Fisac JL et al (2003) A simple estimate of mortality attributable to excess weight in the European Union. *Eur J Clin Nutr* **57**(2): 201–8

Billingham K (2005) Front line framework. *Nurs Stand* **19**(25): 16–7

British Thoracic Society (2006) The Burden of Lung Disease 2006. http://tinyurl.com/4h6mco (accessed 25 September 2009)

Brooker C (2006) *Mosby Nurse's Pocket Dictionary.* 33rd edn. Elsevier Mosby, Edingburgh

Camsooksai J (2002) The role of the Lecturer Practitioner in interprofessional education. *Nurse Educ Today* **22**(6): 466–75

DH (2000) *The NHS Plan: a plan for investment, a plan for reform.* DH, London

DH (2001) *The expert patient: a new approach to chronic disease management for 21st century.* DH, London: ref 2001

DH (2004a) *National Standards Local Action: Health and Social Care Standards and Planning Framework 2005/6–2007/8.* The Stationery Office, London

DH (2004b) Choosing Health: Making healthy choices easier. DH, London: ref 4135

DH (2005a) *Supporting people with long term conditions: Liberating the talents of nurses who care for people with long term conditions.* DH, London: ref 3853

DH (2005b) *Supporting people with long term conditions: An NHS and social care model to support local innovation and integration.* DH, London: ref 4230

DH (2005c) *The National Service Framework for Long-term Conditions.* DH, London: ref 4377

DH (2005d) *Case management competences framework for the care of people with long term conditions.* DH, London: ref 5283

DH (2005e) Public Attitudes to Self Care—Baseline Survey, February 2005. DH, London: ref 4828

DH (2006) *Our health, our care, our say.* DH, London

DH (2008a) *Raising the Profile of Long Term Conditions Care: A Compendium of Information.* DH, London: ref 8734

DH (2008b) *NHS Next Stage Review: Our vision for primary and community care.* DH, London: ref 10096

DH (2008c) *High quality care for all: NHS Next Stage Review final report.* DH, London: ref 10106

DH (2009) *Your health, your way—a guide to long term conditions and self care*. DH, London

Diabetes UK (2009) What is Diabetes? http://tinyurl.com/c7v9k5 (accessed 25 September 2009)

Dixon J, Lewis R, Rosen R, Finlayson B, Gray D (2004) Can the NHS learn from US managed care organisations? *BMJ* **328**(7433): 223–5

Doyle J (2008) Barriers and facilitators of multidisciplinary team working: a review. *Paediatr Nurs* **20**(2): 26–9

Expert Patients Programme Community Interest Company (2007a) Expert Patients Programme. www.expertpatients.co.uk/public/default.aspx (accessed 25 September 2009)

Expert Patients Programme Community Interest Company (2007b) *Self-management of Long-term Health Conditions*. Bull Publishing Company, Colorado

Furze G, Donnison J, Lewin R (2008) *The Clinician's Guide to Chronic Disease Management of Long Term Conditions: A Cognitive Behavioural Approach*. M&K Update Ltd, Cumbria

Gawande A (2007) The bell curve. In: Gawande A. ed, *Better: A Surgeon's Notes on Performance*. Profile Books, London

Glen S (2004) Interprofessional education: the evidence base influencing policy and policy makers. *Nurse Educ Today* **24**(3): 157–9

Griffiths C, Brock A (2003) Twentieth century mortality trends in England and Wales. *Health Stat Q* **18**(summer): 5–18

Hunter M (2005) Eyes shut to social care. *Community Care*. 10 February: 24–5

Hutt R, Rosen R, McCauley J (2004) *Case-managing Long-term Conditions*. The King's Fund, London

Jelphs K, Dickinson H (2008) *Working in Teams*. The Policy Press, Bristol

Koch T, Jenkin P, Kralik D (2004) Chronic illness self-management: locating the 'self'. *J Adv Nurs* **48**(5): 484–92

Masterson A (2007a) Community matrons: promoting self management (part four). *Nurs Older People* **19**(7): 29–32

Masterson A (2007b) Community matrons: inter-professional and inter-agency working (part five). *Nurs Older People* **19**(8): 38–40

Miers M, Pollard K (2009) The role of nurses in interprofessional health and social teams. *Nurs Manag* **15**(9): 30–5

NHS Modernisation Agency (2005) *Good Care Planning for People with Long Term Conditions*. September 2005. Matrix Research Consultancy, London

NHS National Workforce Projects (2006) *Long Term Conditions Case Management*. NHS National Workforce Projects, Manchester

Office for National Statistics (2006) General Household Survey 2005. http://tinyurl.com/ c9pdgd (accessed 25 September 2009)

Office for National Statistics (2008a) National Population Projections. http://tinyurl.com/ yeeon7d (accessed 25 September 2009)

Office for National Statistics (2008b) United Kingdom Health Statistics. http://tinyurl. com/5gjftw (accessed 7 October 2009)

Quality and Outcomes Framework (2006/07) QOF Database Statistics 2006/07. www. gpcontract.co.uk (accessed 25 September 2009)

Roland M, Ducheiko M, Gravelle H, Parker S (2005) Follow up of people aged 65 and over with a history of emergency admission: analysis of routine admission data. *BMJ* **330**(7486): 289–92

Scott H (2004) The matron role is to be developed in the community. *Br J Nurs* **13**(12): 689

The King's Fund (2005) *Patients at Risk of Re-Hospitalisation (PARR) Case Finding Tool.* The King's Fund, London

The King's Fund (2006) *Combined Predictive Model Final Report.* The King's Fund, London

Walsh C, Gordon F, Marshall M, Wilson F, Hunt T (2005) Interprofessional capability: a framework for interprofessional education. *Nurse Educ Pract* **3**: 1–8

Wilson T, Buck D, Ham C (2005) Rising to the challenge: will the NHS support people with long term conditions? *BMJ* **330**(7492): 657–61

World Health Organization (2002) *Reducing risks promoting healthy life.* WHO, Geneva

World Health Organization (2005) Preventing chronic diseases: a vital investment. www. who.int/chp/chronic_disease_report/en/ (accessed 25 September 2009)

World Health Organization (2007) World Health Statistics 2007. www.who.int/whosis/ whostat/2007/en/ (accessed 25 September 2009)

# CHAPTER 2

# Diabetes

*Ruth Rojahn*

This chapter explores the condition of diabetes mellitus, often simply referred to as diabetes. The aim of this chapter is to provide you with an understanding of some of the problems and issues which may affect the life and experiences of the individual with a diagnosis of diabetes. Reading this chapter and reflecting on your own experiences should enable you to achieve the following learning outcomes:

- To review your knowledge of diabetes, and its importance in health care
- To understand the impact of diabetes on lifestyle and quality of life
- To explore the coping mechanisms individuals may use to manage their condition
- To examine the management strategies enabling individuals to manage the long-term effects of diabetes.

## Diabetes mellitus

Diabetes is a metabolic disease primarily characterized by the evidence of abnormally raised blood glucose (hyperglycaemia). Metabolic diseases are those affecting the chemical reactions that occur in the body, which allow growth, reproduction and repair. Diabetes affects the ability of the body to absorb and use glucose as part of the process of nutrition. Glucose metabolism is controlled by a complex interaction of chemicals and hormones, including the hormone insulin, which is produced by the beta cells of the pancreas. Diabetes occurs when there is reduced or absent production of insulin, or when the action of insulin produced is ineffective. Diabetes is classified as being type 1, caused by the failure of the pancreas to produce insulin, and type 2, caused by an inadequate production of insulin or an ineffective use of the insulin that is produced (*Table 2.1*)

Diabetes can also occur in pregnant women and this is called gestational diabetes. The high demands of pregnancy and the growing foetus can sometimes result in an inadequate supply of insulin being produced, which affects the metabolism of glucose in the pregnant woman. Although

**Table 2.1  Differences between type 1 and 2 diabetes**

|  | Type 1 diabetes | Type 2 diabetes |
|---|---|---|
| **Age of onset** | Usually juvenile or young adult onset | Usually middle age or mature onset |
| **Prevalence** | Least common of the two main diabetes types and accounts for only 5–15% of all people with diabetes | More common than type 1 diabetes and accounts for 85–90% of all people with diabetes |
| **Possible cause** | An environmental trigger such as a virus, which may cause an autoimmune attack, preventing the pancreas from producing insulin | Linked to obesity and a sedentary lifestyle |
| **Therapy** | Always requires insulin medication | May be treated by diet and exercise, oral medication and/or insulin |

expectant mothers with diabetes can and do have healthy pregnancies, they are at greater risk of complications, such as needing Caesarean section or contracting infections (Confidential Enquiry into Maternal and Child Health [CEMACH], 2007). They may also develop pre-eclampsia. This is a toxic condition occurring later in the pregnancy that causes a sudden rise in blood pressure, weight gain, and oedema in the hands and legs. Also, babies of women with diabetes are five times more likely to be stillborn (CEMACH, 2007). Gestational diabetes is usually short term and disappears after the baby is born; however, these women are often more at risk of developing type 2 diabetes later in life (NHS Choices, 2009).

## The burden of diabetes

In the UK, the burden of diabetic disease has considerable cost implications for national healthcare expenditure. The aims for services, therefore, should not only be to manage the complications of the disease for patients, but also to consider the implications for policy and practice in light of the cost to the NHS. Diabetes creates a heavy burden for healthcare services and impacts severely on individuals. In order to tackle the disease, one of the most important activities which must be undertaken is to determine the prevalence of diabetes within the community to identify the size and nature of the problem. This has led to the creation of diabetes registers set up by healthcare providers as part of the delivery strategy of the National Service Framework (NSF) (Department of Health [DH], 2003). Communities can have distinct populations, encompassing ethnicity, age and gender range, and levels of deprivation. These factors will determine the specific needs of the local people in order to provide targeted and cost-effective services.

---

### Reflection

Examine your local area and its population. Explore diabetes in relation to the services available in the area provided by:
* Statutory agencies such as local health trusts
* Private agencies such as employers
* Voluntary agencies such as the British Diabetic Association.

---

## Epidemiology

The number of people with diabetes is increasing as a result of global population growth, the ageing population, and the increasing prevalence of obesity and physical inactivity, especially within Western cultures (Kopelman et al, 2005). This has implications for communities with regard to the increased global movement of people, and especially in areas where there are increasing numbers of refugees and asylum seekers. In addition, people of South Asian and African–Caribbean descent have a higher risk of diabetes compared with white European and other ethnic groups. The prevalence of diabetes is higher in men than women, but there are more women with diabetes than men. This is because women live an average of seven years longer than men, and therefore there are more elderly women than men with diabetes.

The most important demographic change to diabetes prevalence across the world appears to be the increase in the proportion of people aged 65 years and older. The prevalence of diabetes for all age groups worldwide was estimated at 2.8% in 2000 and is set to rise to 4.4% in 2030, and the total number of people with diabetes is projected to rise from 171 million in 2000 to 366 million in 2030 (Wild et al, 2004). Therefore, the problem is set to double over the coming years, and given the increasing prevalence of obesity, it is likely that these figures are a conservative estimate of the level of impact that diabetes will have on global health. In addition, there may be many more people who have not yet been diagnosed, who may be unaware that they have the condition, and so are not counted within these numbers. This may be the case especially in type 2 diabetes, the predominant type of diabetes in adults, which accounts for 85–90% of all cases (Department of Health [DH], 2009).

---

**Reflection**

Examine your local area and its population. Explore diabetes in relation to:
- Prevalence and incidence
- Demographic influences on these figures, such as gender, ethnicity or age.

---

## The cost of diabetes

Diabetes places a great burden on both healthcare services and the lives of patients. Approximately 5% of total NHS expenditure, and up to 10% of hospital inpatient costs, is used for the care of people with diabetes (DH, 2007a). The greatest cost of diabetes, however, should be considered in human terms; to the people who have it, their families, carers and friends. The impact of reduced life expectancy and quality of life on these groups is substantial. Life expectancy is reduced, on average, by more than 15 years in people with type 1 diabetes, and between five and seven years in those with type 2 diabetes (at age 55 years). Adults with diabetes have heart disease death rates almost two to four times higher than adults without diabetes, and the risk of stroke is also two to four times higher (DH, 2007a). It is the most common cause of both non-traumatic lower-limb amputation, and end-stage renal disease (DH, 2006a). Hyperglycaemia contributes directly to atherosclerosis by causing endothelial changes in the vascular system. Hyperglycaemia has been shown to cause the glycosylation of proteins, leading to the formation of atheromatous plaques and atherosclerosis (Haffner, 1998). The development of atherosclerosis in arterial circulation impairs blood flow to the distal limbs by reducing the lumen of the affected vessels, which can lead to cell death, necrosis and gangrene, and may require amputation. This means that many individuals are living with a complex mix of diseases, which has an effect on both life expectancy and quality of life. This can range from managing a very healthy lifestyle with the disease, to the extreme of being disabled by diabetic complications and multiple comorbidities. For the latter group, coordinated care which addresses the complex and debilitating problems of multiple morbidity, will be an indication of the quality of life experienced, and those in receipt of well planned care are likely to report better quality of life.

Another factor to be considered is the impact that the disease has on family and carers, who are often relied on to assist in care, or at least be aware of the complications that may arise in the event of a crisis (e.g. hypoglycaemic episodes). This can have an even greater impact if family members do not share the same home, or are some distance away. Support may take the form of helping with shopping and cooking, to the administration of medication and insulin injections. This can become particularly onerous when the condition lasts for many years, and is complicated by distressing complications or deterioration caused by the diseases of old age such as arthritis, dementia or incontinence.

The burden of diabetes also has considerable cost implications for the NHS. This has been estimated to be approximately £1.3 billion per year (Wanless, 2004), much of which is spent on managing the complications caused by the disease. The aims for services, therefore, should be to manage the complications of the disease for patients, as well as to consider the implications for policy and practice in light of the cost to the NHS. The considerations of public demands for value for money, in addition to expectations for scientific innovations to find a cure, create a dilemma for all health professionals.

## The long-term effects of diabetes on individuals

The significance of diabetes for the individual is the effect that a raised blood sugar has on the systems of the body, which results in a range of symptoms and side-effects (*Table 2.2*).

If the condition is left untreated, it can cause a number of long-term problems and ultimately, it can lead to premature death. Therefore a diagnosis of diabetes can be devastating for the patient initially, but will also affect both short- and long-term lifestyle and goals.

Importantly, the impact of a diagnosis of diabetes for an individual means an acceptance of change (there is no cure at present), and once diagnosed, that person will have to live with the condition for the rest of his/her life. The impact that this has at the point of diagnosis may lead to the development of depression, or he/she may undergo a period of grieving for the loss of 'normality', similar to the loss of a loved one identified by Kubler-Ross and Kessler (2005), and may also include feelings of anger and denial.

**Table 2.2 The effects of raised blood sugar on the systems of the body**

| System | Potential long-term effects of diabetic hyperglycaemia |
| --- | --- |
| Sight | Cataract, retinopathy, glaucoma, blindness |
| Skin | Poor healing of wounds, skin infections, peripheral neuropathy |
| Genitourinary | Impotence, urinary tract infections, vaginal yeast infections, nephropathy, renal failure |
| Cardiovascular | Peripheral arterial disease, gangrene, atherosclerosis, stroke, heart attack |
| Gastrointestinal tract | Gum disease, gastroparesis (caused by damage to the vagal nerve) |

**Case study**

*George, aged 54 years, is a lorry driver. He has smoked for most of his adult life, although he has cut down to 15 cigarettes per day. He is frequently away from home as he travels nationwide with his job, and stays away overnight. He sleeps in his cab and uses motorway cafés for meals. He has been diagnosed with type 2 diabetes.*

Consider the following questions in relation to activities such as eating, leisure, travel and work:
- How might diabetes affect George's life?
- What changes might George have to make to his lifestyle?
- How might it affect his life in the long-term?

## Service provision

In the light of the diabetes epidemic, the increasing numbers of people with diabetes will have severe implications for resource management. The DH (2001) recognizes the importance of facilitating individuals to self-manage their long-term conditions as a way of managing the escalating impact that the disease will have on public health as a whole. The NHS has only a finite budget and limited resources and, in order to be cost-effective, emphasis must be placed on encouraging individuals to manage their condition themselves. This style of care moves away from the paternalistic approach evident in the past. The current philosophy is that of supported self-care (DH, 2001). This will be based on a promotional style of health care and includes helping individuals and their families to develop the knowledge and skills to confidently manage their condition. This will require a multi-professional approach, using integrated teams and systematic ongoing support to ensure that the needs of individuals are met in a manner that is specific and seamless.

However, it is important to recognize that individuals have differing needs, depending on where they fall on the continuum between health and disease, and the lifespan continuum and death (*Figure 2.1*).

Therefore, the needs of the diabetic patient will range from none, if he/she is self-caring, to total dependence, if he/she has multiple and complex problems. The needs will also vary depending on the age at which diagnosis is made, as well as the duration of the disease for an individual. The person with diabetes is likely to die on average 20 years earlier than someone without the disease (DH, 2001). Approximately 80% of patients die from the cardiovascular complications of diabetes, as well as being affected by other complications. such as sight problems, and peripheral neuropathy (DH, 2001).

Patients will require varying degrees of intervention in order to maintain and manage the condition effectively. Those with complex needs or multiple conditions may require the intervention of more specialist services to help manage their diabetic care. In some instances, individuals who frequently use unplanned secondary care may require a more intensive and proactive management process to anticipate and preempt such admissions, and to coordinate care from professionals in both health and social care services to ensure a structured, seamless and consistent response. Care for these individuals may fall within the remit of the community matron or other professional, using a case management approach. Whichever style of care is delivered, the aim must always be to maintain or improve the health and quality of life for both individuals and their families and carers.

*Figure 2.1 The health–disease, life–death, birth–death continuum*

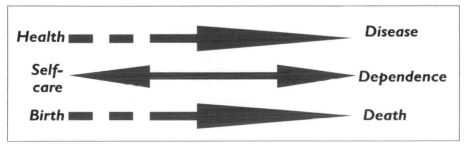

---

**Reflection**

Explore your local services and make a list of the professionals who may input into the care of people with diabetes in the area.
- What is their role?
- How do they contribute to improving the quality of life for the individual, or his/her family?

---

## Health inequalities and national standards

Individuals and their families are an integral part of the larger community, and so it follows that the impact of diabetes will flow into the communities of which they are a part. The health status of a community is a reflection of its differing demographic and epidemiological factors, but this has resulted in unacceptable inequalities, both in levels of health and service provision across communities. Tackling health inequalities has been a high priority for Government since the *Black Report* (Department of Health and Social Security [DHSS], 1980), and current policies have focused on narrowing the health gap between disadvantaged groups, communities and the rest of the country, and on improving the health of the population as a whole (DH, 2006b). To this end, the DH, as part of its review of the NHS, introduced a series of national standards with the aim of reducing inequality and ensuring equitable service provision across all communities. The *National Service Framework for Diabetes* (DH, 2001) set out a series of guidelines for service providers, professionals and communities, which were intended to reduce inequalities, provide evidence-based rationale for effective practice, and increase life expectancy and reduce the risk of complications for people with diabetes in the long term.

The objectives of creating this framework were to empower people to self-manage their condition and encourage them to be involved in decisions about their care. Standard 3, in particular, urges that everyone diagnosed with diabetes should receive a service which encourages partnership in decision-making, supports them in managing their diabetes, and helps them to embrace a healthy lifestyle (DH, 2001: 5). Standards 10, 11 and 12 set out principles which should be adopted by both people with diabetes and those who are involved in their care, to manage the long-term complications that may occur during their lives. The NSF suggests that there is evidence to support the concept that self-management should be the cornerstone for effective care, and improved patient outcomes, but that this will entail effective multi-agency working (DH, 2001).

The standards identify a range of strategies by which the lives of those with diabetes may be improved. The NSF also recommends that the promotion of healthy lifestyles for all by health professionals may help to minimize the long-term effects of diabetes and reduce the risk to the population of developing the disease.

---

### Reflection

- Examine the strategies which health professionals may use with regard to diabetes from a health promotional perspective, in relation to diet, exercise, smoking, work and travel
- Consider which health professionals may be involved in promoting these activities.

---

### National Service Framework for Diabetes: Standards

Standard 1: Prevention of type 2 diabetes
*The NHS will develop, implement and monitor strategies to reduce the risk of developing type 2 diabetes in the population as a whole, and to reduce the inequalities in the risk of developing type 2 diabetes.*
**Implication for practice:** *This will increase the importance of health promotion as a strategy for health professionals. It also places a degree of responsibility on people to lead a healthy lifestyle.*

Standard 2: Identification of people with diabetes
*The NHS will develop, implement and monitor strategies to identify people who do not know they have diabetes.*
**Implication for practice:** *This will increase the need for screening of the population in the community to identify undiagnosed diabetes. Screening processes may have to target people who consider themselves healthy in order to identify the 'hidden' population who are undiagnosed. This may mean the introduction of screening in workplaces and other environments where healthy people can be accessed, and not just in the health service environment.*

Standard 3: Empowering people with diabetes
*All children, young people and adults with diabetes will receive a service which*

encourages partnership in decision-making, supports them in managing their diabetes, and helps them to adopt and maintain a healthy lifestyle. This will be reflected in an agreed and shared care plan. Where appropriate, parents and carers should be fully engaged in this process.

**Implication for practice:** This underlines the need for good communication skills on the part of professionals, and the importance of identifying vulnerable groups and individuals to ensure equity. It also places a degree of significance on the value of community profiling to ensure that minority groups (e.g. the homeless, asylum seekers, children) are not excluded by virtue of their potential inability to articulate their needs.

### Standard 4: Clinical care of adults with diabetes

All adults with diabetes will receive high quality care throughout their lifetime, including support to optimize the control of their blood glucose, blood pressure and other risk factors for developing complications of diabetes.

**Implication for practice:** The importance of evidence-based practice to ensure current treatment is up-to-date and effective is essential to achieve this outcome. It will be necessary to provide accessible and local services to enable availability of this type of ongoing, life-long support.

### Standards 5 and 6: Clinical care of children and young people with diabetes

All children and young people with diabetes will receive consistently high quality care and they, with their families and others involved in their day-to-day care, will be supported to optimize the control of blood glucose and physical, psychological, intellectual, educational and social development.

**Implication for practice:** Promoting self-care for children and young people will help to prevent dependence on the finite resources of the health service through the prevention of long-term complications.

All young people with diabetes will experience a smooth transition of care from paediatric diabetes services to adult diabetes services, whether hospital or community-based, either directly or via a young people's clinic. The transition will be organized in partnership with each individual and at an age appropriate to and agreed with them.

**Implication for practice:** The importance of multi-agency collaboration is essential to ensure this standard. Multi-agency working across children's and adult's services will ensure a seamless transfer of support.

### Standard 7: Management of diabetic emergencies

The NHS will develop, implement and monitor agreed protocols for rapid and effective treatment of diabetic emergencies by appropriately trained health professionals. Protocols will include the management of acute complications and procedures to minimize the risk of recurrence.

*Implication for practice:* People with diabetes and their families should be trained to recognize the onset of diabetic emergencies to access emergency care quickly. The use of telemedicine may enable comprehensive monitoring of glycaemic control and prevent such emergencies.

### Standard 8: Care of people with diabetes during admission to hospital

All children, young people and adults with diabetes admitted to hospital, for whatever reason, will receive effective care of their diabetes. Wherever possible, they will continue to be involved in decisions concerning the management of their diabetes.

*Implication for practice:* Specialist diabetes practitioners will play an important role in supporting other professionals to ensure effective care is given by secondary services. Communication between primary and secondary care will ensure that transfer back into the community is swift and robust.

### Standard 9: Diabetes and pregnancy

The NHS will develop, implement and monitor policies that seek to empower and support women with pre-existing diabetes, and those who develop diabetes during pregnancy to optimize the outcomes of their pregnancy.

*Implication for practice:* Midwives will have a role in supporting women who may have or develop diabetes in pregnancy. Comprehensive assessment processes will play an important part in detecting gestational diabetes, and follow-up care pathways will prevent women being lost from the system following delivery.

### Standards 10, 11 and 12: Detection and management of long-term complications

All young people and adults with diabetes will receive regular surveillance for the long-term complications of diabetes.

The NHS will develop, implement and monitor agreed protocols and systems of care to ensure that all people who develop long-term complications of diabetes receive timely, appropriate and effective investigation and treatment to reduce their risk of disability and premature death.

All people with diabetes requiring multi-agency support will receive integrated health and social care.

*Implication for practice:* Regular health checks should be fair and accessible, which may impact on levels of service provision in the community, with the provision of clinics around family and work commitments. Statutory services may have to work more closely with voluntary services to meet these provisions.

From: DH (2001)

# Management

The management of long-term conditions has become the focus of national policy since the introduction of the *NHS Plan* (DH, 2000), which has led to a different way of managing chronic disease. Two issues have driven this change with regard to diabetes. Firstly, the underpinning philosophy has moved away from a reactive acute-centred model of care to one which is proactive and community-focused. Secondly, there is evidence to support the philosophy that improving the glycaemic control of people with diabetes has significant and positive outcomes both for the individual and for the service providers (Yorkshire and Humber Public Health Observatory, 2006). Patients experience improved quality of life and healthcare services can make significant savings in resources (Wagner et al, 2001). The Government's current strategy for managing long-term conditions has taken three different approaches to diabetes care: case management, disease management, and support for self-management (Hutt et al, 2004). There is growing awareness of the role of peer-led and 'expert patient' interventions to facilitate self-management, particularly to meet the support and informational needs of individuals with long-term conditions. These have been shown to lead to improved clinical outcomes, and relieve pressure on health service providers. There is also increasing interest in telephone support, known as telemedicine, owing to its potential for wide accessibility and availability, rather than the face-to-face support which has been provided to date.

## Case management

Case management comprises the provision of care that is both proactive and individualized for those with complex health and social care needs, through the services of a case manager or a community matron. This group of people will have more than one long-term condition and makes up 3–5% of the UK population (DH, 2004a). This type of care aims to prevent unnecessary admissions to hospital by supporting patients in the community setting with a personalized and coordinated approach. This contributes both to the quality of life for the individual and also for the carers, who may otherwise face having to struggle through a number of different statutory care systems in order to access support and care, or who may be unaware of services in place within their community. The initial activity which must precede case management for diabetes is that of identifying the population at risk. Those risks will include one or more of the following:

- Having two or more long-term conditions relating to diabetes
- Unplanned hospital admissions with an acute diabetic episode

- Frequent appointments with the GP for diabetes-related problems
- Identified as at-risk because of poor disease management quantified by abnormal screening results, such as an abnormal $HbA_{1c}$
- A multiple medication regimen, which may impact on the functional abilities of the patient.

Following the identification of the caseload, the case manager, likely to be the community matron or practice nurse, will undertake a comprehensive assessment for each individual to identify health needs and negotiate a care plan in collaboration with that individual and his/her carers, working closely with other health professionals involved in the case. If the individual has social problems, such as financial difficulties or poor housing, it may also include

---

### Case study

George is an 82-year-old gentleman with type 1 diabetes and arthritis, who lives with his 78-year-old wife, Ethel, who has mild dementia. George is her main carer. They live in a rural community in a large detached house, and their only child, Mary, lives 100 miles away and is still working. George has had several admissions to the local hospital with both hypoglycaemic and hyperglycaemic attacks over the last 18 months as a result of his inability to manage his diet, having taken over the shopping and cooking over the last 2 years since Ethel's dementia has worsened. He now also has problems with his eyesight and is not sure whether he can see the markings on the syringes when he draws up the insulin. He clings to his independence, and is desperate not to seek help as he fears Ethel will be taken away from him and they have been married for nearly 60 years.

His $HbA_{1c}$ results have returned and reflect the poor glycaemic control in George's condition. He has visited the doctor on several occasions in the last few months complaining of not feeling well, that his blood sugar results have been raised, and asking for advice on managing his condition. The GP has increased his insulin medication several times, but this has failed to control his hyperglycaemic attacks.

Consider a case management approach for George in relation to:
- The assessment of his needs—including Ethel in this assessment—taking a holistic and community-focused approach
- The support that George and Ethel may need from both professional and family
- Who is best placed to give this support from the multidisciplinary team?
- The people who will be involved in his care and the information that needs to be communicated to them
- The roles and responsibilities of the case manager in this case.

members of the social care team, such as a district nurse, and GP, as well as any social services providers and voluntary agencies involved in the care.

In the case of pregnant women and children, the health visitor, school nurse or midwife may also be included. Each professional may be involved in the care of a diabetic patient, and the role of the case manager is to act as a coordinator and source of expertise. The case manager will have an enhanced level of knowledge of each individual client relating to the whole range of problems, and therefore will be in a position to recognize deviation from norm, so that any changes can be quickly detected and crisis situations and emergency care averted. There will also be opportunities to review the ongoing care so that changes in treatment can be effected and communicated to all concerned in a timely and effective manner.

## Disease management

The UK Prospective Diabetes Study 10-year post-trial results demonstrated the benefits of early intervention to ensure optimal glycaemic control (Holman et al, 2008). Glycaemic control can be achieved by regulating diet, taking oral anti-hyperglycaemic agents, the administration of subcutaneous injections of insulin, or combination therapy. The choice of therapy will depend on whether the individual has type 1 or type 2 diabetes. Type 1 diabetes will always require insulin. Type 2 may be managed by diet, oral agents, or a combination of both, but may progress to insulin therapy to achieve glycaemic control (*Table 2.1*). Traditionally, the introduction of insulin therapy for type 2 diabetes was often delayed owing to concerns over possible needle phobia or perceived inconvenience to the individual, which may impact on quality of life. In addition, type 2 diabetes was erroneously considered to be a milder form of the disease for which insulin administration was inappropriate (Goldstein and Müller-Wieland, 2007). Many people feared that moving onto insulin medication was an indication that their condition was becoming worse, and it raised anxieties for future wellbeing. Since the introduction of better and more user-friendly administration devices, as well as more effective types of insulin, this practice is now not considered best practice because delay in introducing insulin therapy may lead to poorer clinical outcomes such as the presence of severe micro- and macrovascular complications (Goldstein and Müller-Wieland, 2007).

### Glycaemic control

Glycaemic control can best be measured by taking a sample of venous blood and measuring the glycosylated haemoglobin ($HbA_{1c}$) levels. For a single blood sample, it provides far more revealing information on diabetic glucose management than a fasting blood sugar value. Haemoglobin is a protein with a function to carry oxygen in the blood. As these proteins travel in the bloodstream, they will inevitably come into contact with glucose, which binds to the haemoglobin A. When bonding occurs, the haemoglobin is said to be glycosylated. In the normal lifespan of the red blood cell, glucose molecules join with haemoglobin, forming glycosylated haemoglobin. Once a haemoglobin molecule is glycosylated, it remains that way. In individuals with poorly controlled diabetes, increases in the quantities of these glycosylated haemoglobin compounds are discernable by taking a blood test. The volume of glycosylated haemoglobin in the red cell is evidence of the average level of glucose to which the cell has been exposed during its lifespan. In other words, if there have been excessive levels of glucose in the blood stream, the likelihood of it attaching to haemoglobin and raising the levels of glycosylated haemoglobin present will increase.

The $HbA_{1c}$ level is proportional to average blood glucose concentration over the previous four weeks to three months. Therefore, measuring glycosylated haemoglobin assesses the effectiveness of therapy and the control achieved by monitoring long-term serum glucose regulation, which is more telling than the one-off result obtained from a single fasting blood glucose sample. The significance of this for practice is that it enables professionals to identify individuals who are non-concordant, but who may report that they are adhering to their regimen. Taking a random blood sugar, or even a fasting blood sugar, will only describe how well the individual has managed their glycaemic control over the last few hours. An elevated $HbA_{1c}$ result signifies that control has been poor over a longer period of time, and the individual may require closer monitoring. It is also significant in that a rise in $HbA_{1c}$ levels is closely and proportionately linked to the emergence of complications such as retinopathy and renal disease.

However, the $HbA_{1c}$ reading is an average reading and does not reveal the blood glucose level of one time in particular, but does reveal whether the patient has been concordant with treatment over a period of approximately three months (the lifespan of a red blood cell). The patient may be reluctant to reveal occasional non-adherence to the therapy regimen because he/she may feel he/she has not 'behaved' in a manner acceptable to the health professional. However, this test will give some indication as to whether the patient has been exposed to high levels of glucose during the previous three months and will enable the health professional to explore with the patient any problems which may have caused this. As patients are being encouraged to self-manage, there is less opportunity for the professional to monitor blood glucose levels more frequently, although patients should be encouraged to test their own blood glucose levels, especially if they feel unwell, and record these to discuss with the professional at an appointment.

The significance of achieving glycaemic control relies on the understanding of the individual to control the nutritional balance required to achieve optimum levels. The role of the dietician is important, to make sure that information about diet is given in understandable and practical terms. To supplement this support and to facilitate dietary control, individuals are encouraged to maintain monitoring diaries. Singh and Press (2008) suggest that the use of a monitoring diary can help to achieve better glycaemic control. A diary will help individuals to record their intake alongside the recorded blood sugar levels, and reflect on both the quality and quantity of nutritional intake. This helps to reinforce the association between carbohydrates and fats with the levels of insulin required. The diary will include information about the individual in relation to medication and diet, as well as keeping a record of blood glucose levels. It may suggest a target range for the blood glucose and $HbA_{1c}$ levels, and identify any key events which may have affected a changed blood level, such as illness, a meal out, or extra physical activity.

Nurses have an important role in the education, promotion of self-care, acquisition of skills, and psychological support for people with life-changing conditions like diabetes. This will require the nurse to have excellent communication and assessment skills in order to gain an insight into any specific needs of patients. Compilation of baseline information from an accurate assessment will enable the nurse to formulate a plan of care which is specific, achievable and meaningful to the patient, which will facilitate patient concordance. Facilitating independence and self-management in diabetic care will depend on the quality of education that patients receive, both at the time of diagnosis and thereafter.

## DESMOND and DAfNE

Diabetes Education and Self-Management for Ongoing and Newly Diagnosed (DESMOND) is a national education programme for people with type 2 diabetes, providing:

- Six hours of group education following a structured programme, either as a one-day course, or as two half-day courses—the two half-days being no more than two weeks apart
- Groups consist of 6–10 people newly diagnosed with type 2 diabetes who can choose to be accompanied by a partner, family member or friend
- Each person attending a group is also provided with information to accompany the programme and intended as a reference guide subsequent to attending the course.

A National Institute for Health and Clinical Excellence (NICE) study (2003) on the use of patient education models for diabetes found that most people with diabetes in England and Wales are offered education, at least at the time of diagnosis. However, it also noted that the length, content and style of educational options varied between services. It found that many educational programmes lacked structure, few were formally evaluated, and many of the facilitators had not received any formal training to deliver such programmes. The study update states that:

*'Management of diabetes typically involves a considerable element of self-care, and advice should, therefore, be aligned with the perceived needs and preferences of people with diabetes, and carers. People with type 2 diabetes should have the opportunity to make informed decisions about their care and treatment, in partnership with their healthcare professionals.'*

*National Institute for Health and Clinical Excellence (2008: 6)*

Loveman et al (2008) conclude that:

*'...education delivered by a team of educators, with some degree of reinforcement of that education made at additional points of contact, may provide the best opportunity for improvements in patient outcomes. Educators need to have time and resources to fulfil the needs of any structured educational programme. There is also a need for education to have a clear programme at the outset.'*

*Loveman et al (2008: 3)*

DESMOND has DH backing, and meets the standards laid down in the NSF for diabetes (DH, 2001) and NICE guidelines (2008). However, DESMOND also provides other direct benefits:

- Provides patients with a good start in the self-management of diabetes
- Empowers patients to self-manage by addressing issues of the initiation and sustaining motivation
- Promotes effective partnerships between primary and specialist services.

The condition and treatment of diabetes has a negative impact on quality of life, particularly in relation to the dietary restrictions imposed by traditional rigid insulin treatment regimens. Adhering to a rigid regimen of eating and administering insulin can restrict an individual's lifestyle choices and activities, which may be reported as being a negative aspect of diabetic care. The Dose Adjustment for Normal Eating (DAfNE) programme suggests an approach in which intensive insulin management is used to increase dietary choice, which is likely to improve quality of life as well as disease outcomes. This is a five-day course onto which small groups of type 1 diabetic patients are enrolled, in order to learn how to take control of the disease and achieve greater freedom of choice in their diet. The emphasis on nutrition is to teach patients to count carbohydrates so that when they have decided what food they would like to eat, they can choose an appropriate insulin dose. The sessions focus on a variety of social situations that may require estimating the amount of carbohydrate there may be in a meal. One carbohydrate portion is roughly equivalent to 10–12 g of carbohydrates. This enables participants to estimate the carbohydrate content of whatever they want to eat, rather than to restrict them to a prescribed diet. Diabetic control is then achieved by adjusting multiple insulin doses in relation to what is eaten, rather than adjusting diet against a set insulin regimen.

The theme of the DAfNE course is 'eat what you like, like what you eat'. This element of management is further explored by Bergenstal et al (2008) who concluded that individuals can learn to adjust their doses of insulin in relation to their nutritional intake, and therefore achieve better glycaemic control, either by using a simple algorithm or learning to use insulin : carbohydrate ratios. They suggest that insulin : carbohydrate ratios allow for greater flexibility in food choices and make relatively precise matching of insulin to meal choices possible. This may not be applicable for all individuals as it can seem complex and difficult to manage. Individuals with poor memory, confusion or lower levels of cognition may have particular problems with this style of management. However, DAfNE training has been shown to significantly improve glycosylated haemoglobin, with no significant increase in severe hypoglycaemia. The training has also produced sustained positive effects on quality of life, satisfaction with treatment, and psychological wellbeing. This is despite an increase in the number of insulin injections and encouragement to increase blood glucose monitoring and therefore the additional burden that this will entail in terms of both time and 'sharps' tasks (DAfNE Study Group, 2002). The success of such programmes, the first of which began in Germany, has been evaluated positively and adopted in other countries, including the UK and Australia. Nevertheless, some professionals have reservations about such a programme and conclude that further research is required (McIntyre, 2006). Compliance with intensive regimens is notoriously difficult in young patients, and the programme does not necessarily include education on healthy eating as part of a health lifestyle advocated in Government policy, for example *Choosing Health* (DH, 2004b).

## Self-management

There is now recognition of the value of knowledge and experience inherent in being an individual with diabetes, which can be channelled into peer support (DH, 2007b). The role of the patient in self-management has extended further than just being encouraged to take responsibility for their own care, and has also moved to taking on the role of educator. In recent years, the importance of developing this role has been promoted by health policy. The *Expert Patient Programme* (DH, 2007b) identifies the ability of patients to successfully guide other patients in becoming 'expert' in their own care, and highlights the value of patient knowledge as an educational and communicative tool (*Table 2.3*).

In view of the expected rise in levels of diabetes both nationally and globally, and the increasing budgetary constraints on service provision, the use of the *Expert Patient Programme* for diabetes provides an opportunity to use a resource which has shown to be both effective and beneficial for all involved. Plews (2005) identifies this as a potentially efficacious, cost-effective and patient-centred method of enhancing self-management. Self management approaches in diabetes improve knowledge, performance of self-management behaviours, self-efficacy and health status, including a reduction in blood glucose levels, calorific intake, weight, and lowering serum cholesterol (Barlow et al, 2001).

In order to enable individuals to self-manage their diabetes, a comprehensive assessment of needs should be undertaken, which should include factors specifically relevant to diabetic disease or which may indicate the presence of diabetic complications (*Table 2.4*). Assessment will provide a baseline of information for ongoing review. It may also give some indication

---

### Table 2.3 The positive effects of the Expert Patient Programme

- Feel confident and in control of their lives
- Aim to manage their condition and its treatment in partnership with health professionals
- Communicate effectively with professionals and are willing to share responsibility and treatment
- Are realistic about the impact of their disease on themselves and their family
- Use their skills and knowledge to lead full lives.

From: DH (2007b)

---

**Table 2.4 Assessment of factors specific to diabetes**

---

- Blood pressure, angina, shortness of breath, dizziness
- Urinalysis
- Fasting blood sugar, $HbA_{1c}$
- A range of blood tests for renal function and cholesterol
- Skills assessment, manual dexterity, cognitive function, sight
- Foot assessment, including vibration sense and peripheral pulses
- Transient weakness, claudication in lower limbs, mobility
- Smoking or tobacco habits
- Dietary habits/preferences
- Exercise/activity habits
- Coping mechanisms, knowledge, beliefs, attitudes

---

as to the current stage of the disease, as the individual may have unknowingly had diabetes for some time before diagnosis, and may already exhibit some of the complications that treatment aims to prevent.

Assessment will include key measurements to determine the levels of glycaemic control achieved. Optimal levels are shown in *Table 2.5*. Variations outside of these ranges will help to identify the development of any cardiovascular, neuropathic or renal complications.

If individuals are to be self-caring, it is essential to ensure that they have not only the physical resources to do so, but also the cognitive and psychological abilities. The benefits of self-management will only be

---

**Table 2.5 Suggested goals of treatment regimen: key measurements**

---

| | |
|---|---|
| $HbA_{1c}$ | < 6.5 mmol/litre |
| Blood pressure | < 130/80 mmHg |
| Total Cholesterol | < 5.0 mmol/l |
| HDL (high-density lipoprotein) | < 1.2 mmol/l |
| LDL (low density lipoprotein) | < 3.0 mmol/l |
| Triglycerides | < 1.7 mmol/l |
| Glucose | 3.3–11 mmol/l |
| Albumin/creatinine ratio (ACR) | < 2.5 mmol/l in men |
| | < 3.5 mmol/l in women |

From: NICE (2008)

---

evident if assessment shows that the individual is truly able to manage the disease, and not merely as a way of reducing costs to healthcare services. It is important to remember that people with diabetes will often have other concomitant disease and may also be elderly. Managing the effects of one disease can be a difficult and time-consuming process, but managing comorbidity is even more complex and requires a higher level of both physical and psychological skills. These factors will impact on the ability of individuals to be self-managing, and it is therefore essential to undertake a thorough assessment of abilities and deficits. It is also important to include a review of the individual's living environment in the assessment, as well as the supporting network of family and carers to address any needs. It has been identified that these factors may significantly contribute to whether an individual can maintain self-care over the duration of a long-term illness like diabetes.

Managing diabetes requires individuals and/or their carers to be able and willing to:

* See sufficiently well to self-medicate, either with oral medications or with injections of insulin. Can they read the label on the medicine bottle/see the marks on an insulin syringe?
* Take their medication and test their blood sugar. Do they have the cognitive abilities to understand the implications of not taking their medication? Do they have enough manual dexterity to open a tablet bottle/draw up insulin in a syringe/load a pen device with needle and cartridge/use a lancet and see the result on the monitoring device?
* Select and prepare a well-balanced and appropriate diet/meal. Can they shop for food/prepare and cook well-balanced meals/eat the food that is prepared?
* Recognize a hypoglycaemic and hyperglycaemic episode and take appropriate action. Can they make decisions with regard to if and when to take bolus glucose or insulin to achieve optimal glycaemic balance?
* Understand what is required for glycaemic control. Do they have sufficient cognitive skills and insight into how to regulate their diet and balance it with the prescribed medication?
* Demonstrate awareness of long-term complications. Do they know how to look after their feet, skin, attend regular check-ups for eye problems, etc?

It is also important to consider the environment and living conditions that may impact on an individual with diabetes. This may include assessing activities of everyday living. A person with diabetes may have the long-term complication of peripheral neuropathy and have reduced feeling in his/her extremities. If the home environment is crowded for example, the individual is at risk of knocking his/her legs on furniture, leading to lacerations and abrasions. An individual with peripheral neuropathy may scald him/herself if bathing in water that is too hot, or may tread on an object and cause a stab wound to the foot. In the case of a person with diabetes, this could lead to wounds which take longer to heal, become infected or ultimately lead to gangrene and amputation of the limb. If the individual has developed sight problems, it may impact on his/her ability to see to prepare food or to maintain the cleanliness of the home, which may make them more susceptible to infection. It is also important to also consider the comorbidities of other diseases, such as arthritis and heart disease, which may impact on mobility and dexterity within the home environment.

The psychological impact of diabetes must also be considered. The impact of diagnosis and prognosis can be considerable and lead to the development of anxiety and depression. Major depression in diabetes has been associated with poor self-care in areas that are difficult to maintain, such as exercise, diet, and medication management. Depression has been shown to lead to poor adherence to medication, lack of glycaemic monitoring, and lack of physical activity (Whiting et al, 2006). Depression may also result in behaviour such as comfort eating, smoking or alcohol use, which has direct impact on the progression of diabetic disease. Individuals who have multiple complex needs owing to the presence of comorbidities may also be at increased risk of depressive episodes. Therefore, better identification and care of depression among people with diabetes may be of benefit not only to improve quality of life of individuals, but also lead to more effective self-management.

Self-management of diabetic disease has been found to be time-consuming for individuals. Russell et al (2005) suggested that self-care involves a range of activities surplus to the normal activities of living, which must be undertaken to effectively manage the condition. These can include glucose monitoring, record-keeping, taking medication, foot care, telephoning health professionals, arranging and attending hospital or clinic appointments, arranging specific insurance, and obtaining supplies. Frequent access to health care, to attend clinics, for monitoring purposes or for treatments, disrupts lifestyle. This extra activity emphasizes the existence of the disease to an individual who is trying to normalize life as part of the underlying philosophy of self-management. These extra tasks may result in the individual being reluctant to take on self-management, or even to deny the reality and impact that having diabetes has on their lives. Such denial may lead to a negative reaction to the management of the disease, and a lack of commitment required to maintain effective control.

# The future

Diabetes is a growing problem on a global scale, and will continue to challenge health professionals over the next few decades in a number of ways. These range from improving provision of care to health promotion and patient education of self care, as well as managing services efficiently and effectively to reduce inequalities and increase quality of life. Sedentary lifestyles and the dependence on vehicular travel, as well as increasing globalization of populations, may lead to increasing levels of obesity and other risk factors for diabetes. In addition, careful profiling and monitoring of communities and increased public education may raise the profile and awareness of the symptoms of diabetes, leading to more people being diagnosed with the condition, especially at an early stage to avoid or delay the onset on complications. Conversely, new technologies and advances in treatments, including innovative mechanical devices to administer insulin and pancreatic transplants, will enable people with diabetes to maintain better glycaemic controls and live longer lives, relatively free from the complications which have hitherto impacted on quality of life. This may, in turn, increase the numbers of diabetic people requiring care, and also result in an increase in the number of diabetics living to an older age who may require care because of conditions affected by ageing. Health professionals will therefore require improved health promotional and educational skills to facilitate support and optimize self-care. Certainly over the last few decades, new approaches to management have led to increased quality of life for diabetics and the knowledge base for practice has grown and is supported by reliable evidence. It is now recognized that this should include the management of cardiovascular risk factors, as well as the implications on the mental health of those with diabetes. The use of telemedicine and the internet will change the traditional ways in which professionals communicate with patients, and may enable them to be less dependent on acute services. But until a cure can be found, the challenge to health professionals will be to both identify and meet the needs of people who may be at risk of diabetes, and also support and educate those who develop the condition.

Barlow J, Wright C, Sheasby J et al (2001) Self-management approaches for people with chronic conditions: a review. *Patient Educ Couns* 48(2): 177–87

Bergenstal R, Johnson M, Powers M et al (2008) Adjust to target in type 2 diabetes: comparison of a simple algorithm with carbohydrate counting for adjustment of mealtime insulin glulisine. *Diabetes Care* 31(7): 1305–10

Confidential Enquiry into Maternal and Child Health (2007) Diabetes in pregnancy: Are we providing the best care? http://tinyurl.com/yfnuota (accessed 26 October 2009)

DAFNE Study Group (2002) Training in flexible, intensive insulin management to enable dietary freedom in people with type 1 diabetes: dose adjustment for normal eating (DAFNE) randomised controlled trial. *BMJ* **325**(7367): 746

DH (2000) *The NHS Plan: a plan for investment, a plan for reform.* DH, London.

DH (2001) *National Service Framework for Diabetes.* DH, London

DH (2003) *National Service Framework for Diabetes: Delivery Strategy.* DH, London. ref: 2003

DH (2004a) *Chronic Disease Management: A compendium of information.* DH, London

DH (2004b) *Choosing Health: Making healthy choices easier.* DH, London. ref: 4135

DH (2006a) *Turning the corner: improving diabetes care.* DH, London. ref: 6421

DH (2006b) *Health Challenge England: Next steps for Choosing Health.* DH, London. ref: 7175

DOH (2007a) *The way ahead: The local challenge.* DH, London. ref: 2915

DH (2007b) *Improving diabetes services: The National Service Framework four years on. The way ahead, the local challenge.* DH, London. ref: 7915

DH (2007c) *The Expert Patients Programme.* DH, London

DH (2009) About diabetes. http://tinyurl.com/ln4nx6 (accessed 26 October 2009)

DHSS (1980) *Inequalities in health: report of a research working group.* DHSS, London

Goldstein BJ, Müller-Wieland D (2007) *Type 2 Diabetes: Principles and Practice.* 2nd edn. Informa Healthcare, London

Haffner SM (1998) Management of dyslipidemia in adults with diabetes. *Diabetes Care* **21**(1): 160–78

Holman RR, Paul SK, Bethel MA, Neil HAW, Matthews DR (2008) UK PDS 10-year follow-up of intensive glucose control in type 2 diabetes. *N Engl J Med* **359**(15): 1565–76

Hutt R, Rosen R, McCauley J (2004) *Case managing long term conditions: what impact does it have in the treatment of older people?* The King's Fund, London

Kopelman PG, Caterson ID, Dietz WH (2005) *Clinical Obesity in Adults and Children.* 2nd edn. Blackwell Publishing Ltd, London

Kubler-Ross E, Kessler D (2005) *On Grief and Grieving: Finding the Meaning of Grief Through the Five Stages of Loss.* Simon & Schuster Ltd, London

Loveman E, Frampton GK, Clegg AJ (2008) The clinical effectiveness of diabetes education models for Type 2 diabetes: a systematic review. Executive Summary. www.ncchta.org/pdfexecs/summ1209.pdf (accessed 1 October 2009)

McIntyre HD (2006) DAFNE (Dose Adjustment for Normal Eating): structured education in insulin replacement therapy for type 1 diabetes. *Med J Aust* **184**(7): 317–8

NHS Choices (2009) Diabetes, type 2. http://tinyurl.com/yfhlln2 (accessed 26 October 2009)

NICE (2003) Diabetes (types 1 and 2)—patient education models. http://guidance.nice.org.uk/TA60 (accessed 1 October 2009)

NICE (2008) Type 2 diabetes: the management of type 2 diabetes. http://guidance.nice.org.uk/CG66 (accessed 1 October 2009)

Russell LB, Suh DC, Safford MA (2005) Time requirements for diabetes self-management: too much for many? *J Fam Pract* **54**(1): 52–6

Singh R, Press M (2008) Can we predict future improvement in glycaemic control? *Diabet Med* **25**(2): 170–3

Wagner EH, Austin BT, Davis C et al (2001) Improving chronic illness care: translating evidence into action. *Health Aff* **20**(6): 64–78

Wanless D (2004) Securing good health for the whole population: Final report. DH, London. ref: 2004

Whiting M, Scammell A, Gray J, Schepers AK, Bifulco A (2006) Managing type 2 diabetes and depression in primary care. *Primary Care Mental Health* **4**(3): 175-184

Wild S, Roglic G, Green A, Sicree R, King H (2004) Global Prevalence of Diabetes. Estimates for the year 2000 and projections for 2030. *Diabetes Care* **27**: 1047–53

Yorkshire and Humber Public Health Observatory (2006) *Diabetes Key Facts.* YHPHO, York

## Useful websites

*DAfNE: www.dafne.uk.com*

*DESMOND: www.desmond-project.org.uk*

*Diabetes UK: www.diabetes.org.uk*

# CHAPTER 3

# Heart failure

*Ruth Rojahn*

Heart failure is a chronic disabling disease, which worsens over time and shortens life expectancy. The aim of this chapter is to explore some of the problems which may affect the life and experiences of the individual with heart failure to enable you to gain some insight into some of the issues surrounding this condition. Reading this chapter and reflecting on your own experiences should enable you to achieve the following learning outcomes:

* To review your knowledge of heart failure and its importance
  in health care
* To understand the impact of heart failure on lifestyle and quality of life
* To explore the coping mechanisms individuals may use to manage
  heart failure
* To examine the management strategies enabling individuals to cope
  with the long-term effects of heart failure.

## Background

In order to understand how heart failure can impact on a person's life, it is important to have an understanding of the condition. Although it can be immediately life-threatening, the long-term outlook will vary from patient to patient, and can depend on age, the severity of the symptoms, and the overall health of the individual. In general, however, the severity of the symptoms are in some measure relative to the estimated lifespan, as they will become more severe as the condition develops, and this will be reflected in the individuals' ability to cope. Therefore, patients will require more input from professionals as the condition progresses.

Heart failure can be extremely debilitating, and the Healthcare Commission (now Care Quality Commission) (2007) states that people with heart failure have a much worse quality of life than those with most other chronic conditions, with over a third experiencing severe and prolonged depressive illness. Heart failure can be both acute and chronic, but for the purposes of this chapter, we shall only consider chronic heart failure as a long-term condition. Chronic heart failure is a long-standing condition occurring over a period of months and years that is associated with the heart undergoing adaptive responses, such as dilation and hypertrophy, from a precipitating cause. If left untreated, it is a serious condition that can result in death quite quickly, so early diagnosis and treatment will enable the individual to extend a potentially poor prognosis. Despite this, by the time heart failure is diagnosed, the individual will already have developed some deficiency in the heart mechanism, which will be evidenced by changes in the physiology of the circulatory system, as well as other bodily systems.

## Causes of chronic heart failure

Lifestyle factors that cause tissue damage, such as alcohol and drug misuse, stress, smoking and a high cholesterol diet, may lead to heart failure, but there are also some unavoidable conditions that can cause the condition. Diseases which affect the valves of the heart and congenital heart defects, as well as atrial fibrillation, place increased demands on the heart and precipitate failure. Heart failure can be caused by intrinsic cardiac factors, originating from within the heart itself. One of the most important causes of heart failure is coronary artery disease, which reduces blood flow to the heart muscle, the myocardium. Another intrinsic factor which may lead to heart failure is myocardial infarction. This is a condition of prolonged ischemia/hypoxia of the myocardium resulting in a reperfusion-induced injury, which causes irreversible damage to the heart muscle. Heart failure can also be caused by extrinsic cardiac factors, which are other external conditions that place excessive demands on the heart and require it to work harder. Some of the extrinsic factors which may lead to heart failure are pregnancy, anaemia, some hormonal conditions such as diabetes and hyperthyroidism, and, most importantly, prolonged and uncontrolled hypertension.

## Heart function

The primary function of the heart is to pump blood around the body, and to do this it must generate and sustain an arterial blood pressure sufficient to provide adequate perfusion of the organs. The heart succeeds in this activity by contracting its muscular walls, the myocardium, to create enough pressure to drive blood from the left ventricle, through the aortic valve, into the aorta and around the body. In order to maintain efficient blood circulation, where there are factors which impact on the heart rate and its ability to maintain the blood circulation, the normal heart physiology will undergo changes. Reviewing knowledge of the normal heart, its anatomy and physiology will enable you to understand the impact that changes which occur in heart failure have on the body systems. To summarize briefly, the changes in cardiac function associated with heart failure result in a decrease in cardiac output, the volume of blood pumped by the heart over one minute. This is a result of a decline in stroke volume owing to systolic dysfunction, diastolic dysfunction, or a combination of the two. Stroke volume is the amount of blood pumped by the left ventricle of the heart in one contraction. Normally, only approximately two thirds of the blood in the ventricle is propelled out with each beat, meaning that the stroke volume is not all of the blood in the left ventricle. The amount of blood that is actually pumped from the left ventricle is the stroke volume and it, together with the heart rate, determines the cardiac output; that is, the output of blood by the heart per minute. Therefore, the result of the heart having to work harder is that it may precipitate physiological adaptions caused by compensatory mechanisms, which occur in order to maintain cardiac output. It is these adaptions and the subsequent resulting organic impact which, if prolonged, will ultimately lead to heart failure and potentially cause death. Therapeutic interventions to improve cardiac output in heart failure include the use of drugs which stimulate the heart muscle and contractility, and regulate the heart rate, as well as vasodilator drugs to produce dilation, and reduce the arterial pressure so that the ventricle can eject blood more rapidly, and therefore enhance stroke volume.

Vasodilator drugs produce dilation, and reduce the arterial pressure so that the ventricle can eject blood more rapidly, and therefore enhance stroke volume. One of the most important types of drugs are ACE inhibitors (angiotensin-converting enzyme inhibitors). They are a type of vasodilator, which cause the blood vessels to expand, lowering blood pressure and reducing the heart's workload, and ultimately slowing the progression of heart failure. ACE inhibitors prevent the body from creating angiotensin, a substance in the blood that causes vessels to tighten and raises blood pressure. Commonly used ACE inhibitors are ramipril, lisinopril, captopril, enalapril and perindopril (Joint Formulary Committee, 2009).

Other medications can be those which stimulate the heart muscle and contractility, and regulate the heart rate, such as beta-blockers. Beta-blockers reduce the heart beat. The drugs block specific receptors (beta receptors) on the cells of heart tissue, reducing the effects of chemical messengers that increase heart rate. This allows the heart to maintain a slower rate and lowers blood pressure. Commonly used beta-blockers are metoprolol, atenolol, bisoprolol, propranolol and acebutolol (Joint Formulary Committee, 2009).

---

**Reflection**

- Review your knowledge of the medications which affect the working of the heart in more detail
- Consider how it might affect the individual with heart failure from a physical and psychological point of view.

---

## Cardiac changes

By the time an individual is diagnosed with chronic heart failure, the heart will have already lost some of its ability to pump blood effectively. Even before symptoms are experienced, the heart has usually been compensating for the inefficient cardiac output. This will result in:

- Enlarging. This increases the capacity of the ventricles, the chambers of the heart, which in turn increases the stroke volume
- Developing more muscle mass. The cardiac muscle cells cause the contractions to increase, allowing the heart to contract more strongly and pump more blood
- Pumping faster. This allows the heart to increase the amount of blood being pumped around the body.

When an individual develops heart failure, the rest of the body may compensate by:

- Narrowing the blood vessels. This raises blood pressure to make up for the loss of power from the heart, to help maintain perfusion of the organs
- Diverting blood. The body diverts blood from less important parts of the body, such as the hands and feet, so that it mostly flows to the vital organs, including the heart and brain.

Although they do not resolve the primary cause, these compensatory measures help with circulation in the initial stages of heart failure. However, it is because of these actions that many people may not be aware that they have heart failure for some years, by which time the condition has progressed to the point where symptoms cause problems and are irreversible.

## Symptoms of heart failure

Heart failure causes a collection of symptoms owing to the reduction in the heart's ability to pump blood around the body. This results in:

- Pulmonary oedema—blood and fluid building up in the lungs and causing persistent coughing or wheezing, and possibly the production of white or pink frothy phlegm
- Distal oedema—a build up of fluid in the abdomen, or in the legs and feet, sometimes leading to cellulitis or leg ulcers
- Lethargy—tiredness and lack of energy
- Anorexia—loss of appetite or nausea
- Weight increase (because of extra fluid in the body) or weight-loss (because of a lack of appetite)
- Dyspnoea—shortness of breath owing to the poor oxygenation of pulmonary blood and the pulmonary oedema
- Lack of sleep—difficulty breathing while lying flat
- Confusion, impaired thinking, memory loss or disorientation
- Palpitations—increased heart rate.

The symptoms of heart failure will depend on whether it occurs on the right or left side of the heart. There may be a mixture of the two if the whole heart is affected. *Tables 3.1* and *3.2* summarize the symptoms which may occur, linked to the causative physiological factors.

These symptoms can be assessed to identify their extent and severity, and classify how much they are affecting the life of the individual. A commonly used assessment tool is the New York Heart Association Functional Classification of Heart Failure symptoms (*Table 3.3*). Walking distance ability may also be used, but this does not correlate with accurately measured exercise capacity owing to variable patient perception of distance, and has been found to have little prognostic relevance. Its value is therefore doubtful.

## Epidemiology

Recent epidemiology of heart failure shows it is a common clinical problem, and affects around 900 000 people in the UK (Healthcare Commission, 2007). It is particularly common among older people, with prevalence expected to increase over the next 20 years (Healthcare Commission, 2007). As previously identified, prognosis from heart failure is poor. Some data has suggested that around 40% of people die within one year of an initial diagnosis of heart failure

**Table 3.1 The symptoms of left-sided heart failure result from congestion of the lungs and reduced cardiac output**

| Symptom | Cause |
|---|---|
| Dyspnoea Orthopnoea Paroxysmal nocturnal dyspnoea | Fluid in the alveoli |
| Cough | Large amounts of frothy blood tinged sputum May be unproductive |
| Altered renal function Oedema Weight gain | Decreased renal blood flow and increased sodium and water reabsorption |
| Anxiety Restlessness Irritability | Cerebral anoxia |
| Fatigue Muscular weakness | Low cardiac output, and impaired oxygenation of tissues and removal of metabolic wastes |

From: Peattie and Walker (1995)

**Table 3.2 The symptoms of right-sided heart failure result from venous congestion of the viscera and peripheral tissues**

| Symptom | Cause |
|---|---|
| Oedema—usually pitting Weight gain Distended neck veins | Venous congestion—impaired sodium excretion |
| Coolness of extremities | Decreased peripheral blood flow owing to venous congestion |
| Abdominal pain Liver enlargement | Hepatic congestion with venous blood |
| Anorexia | |
| Nausea abdominal organs | Venous engorgement and stasis within |
| Anxiety Fear | Symptoms and the condition |

From: Peattie and Walker (1995)

**Table 3.3 New York Heart Association Functional Classification of Heart Failure symptoms**

| | |
|---|---|
| **Class I** | No limitation of physical activity. Ordinary activity does not cause undue fatigue or breathlessness |
| **Class II** | Slight limitation of physical activity. Comfortable at rest, but ordinary physical activity results in fatigue or breathlessness |
| **Class III** | Marked limitation of physical activity. Comfortable at rest, but less than ordinary activity causes fatigue or breathlessness |
| **Class IV** | Unable to carry out any physical activity without symptoms. Symptoms are present even at rest. If any physical activity is undertaken, symptoms are increased |

From: Raphael et al (2007)

(Cowie et al, 2000). A quarter die within three months, over a third by one year, and nearly one in two patients are dead by two years (Cowie et al, 2000). Most deaths within the first three months occur during the first admission to hospital, and this ominous prospect is regardless of the interventions of current therapies (Wood, 2002). In effect, the individual with heart failure is given a death sentence and must come to terms with the fact that his/her life expectancy has been cut short. Combining data on incidence and survival, estimates in 2001 suggested that the number of deaths from heart failure in the UK was at least 24 000 (British Heart Foundation (BHF), 2006). This means at least 4% of all deaths in the UK are a result of heart failure (BHF, 2006). This, and the expected increase in the mortality rate, will affect how health and social care services use future resources to support those groups affected by the condition. Cowie (2001) reports that women may have a lower mortality rate than men because at the same chronological age, a woman's body is biologically younger than a man's and more able to cope with the development of poor pump function, although the data may have inherent bias which has affected the results of the research (Cowie et al, 2000).

**Reflection**

- Explore the data for your local area in relation to morbidity and mortality
- Consider how this may reflect the needs of the local population
- Compare your findings with national data and analyse why there may be differences.

# The impact of heart failure on service provision

The growing numbers of elderly within the population, as well as the increasing incidence of heart failure owing to current lifestyle practices, especially in the Western world, means that providing an efficient and effective heart failure service is paramount if finite NHS resources are to meet the needs of the population it serves. In addition, if a previously unidentified excessive demand for diagnosis and care emerges, it could have adverse implications on the capacity of services to deal with extra demand, the costs of prescribing, and the length of waiting times (Healthcare Commission, 2007).

Heart failure accounts for about 5% of all medical admissions to hospital and those with the condition are frequently readmitted to hospital. In fact, readmission rates for heart failure are among the highest for any common condition in the UK and have been estimated to be as high as 50% over three months—approximately half of these admissions may be preventable (Department of Health [DH], 2000). This is referred to as the 'revolving door' factor. Recent developments in risk-predictive tools are enabling primary care trusts (PCTs) to direct resources more accurately to reduce readmissions. The development of the Patients at Risk of Re-admission (PARR) tool was originally commissioned by the DH, alongside the agenda to develop community matron teams (The King's Fund, 2009). The aim was to clarify which patients are most at risk of readmission, using inpatient data to manage long-term conditions in the community and cut revolving-door admissions. However, while identifying patients at risk is necessary and valid, the real key to reducing recurrent admissions is the development of clinically effective interventions.

While the PARR tool is helpful in identifying patients at risk, it does not currently calculate the reduction in acute admissions in real terms. There are now other risk-prediction tools on the market, but currently PARR remains the only one that is free for NHS trusts. A King's Fund survey showed that 60% of PCTs are using the PARR tool (Hunt, 2008).

The potential advantages of an efficient heart failure service with effective clinical interventions, as part of an NHS providing better care for the treatment of people with chronic heart failure are:

*   Early diagnosis and effective evidence-based treatment will enable both prolonged life, and improved quality of life and management of the disease for individuals and their families
*   By reducing the progression rate of the condition so that individuals stay well for longer, clinical outcomes will be improved

- Enabling individuals to stay at home by providing specialist care coordinated between primary and secondary care will reduce hospital stay for individuals with chronic heart failure and prevent 'revolving door' admissions
- Increasing and enabling patient choice by holistic assessment, a joined-up approach to care, and optimizing their management plan and communicating effectively with the primary care team, patient and carers
- Reducing inequalities within communities by improving equality of access to diagnosis and treatment, and setting national standards for clinical care
- Improving knowledge of heart failure among ethnic and other vulnerable and minority groups, and targeting high-risk groups to facilitate clinical outcomes
- Better value for money and efficient use of resources by community profiling, which will help to target services efficiently and meet local need.

This requires a multi-professional approach to ensure that appropriate referral pathways are in place and that the multidisciplinary specialist heart failure service is integrated with other services, including primary, secondary and social care.

In the *National Service Framework for Coronary Heart Disease* (DH, 2000), Standard 11 suggested that the NHS should, when caring for patients with heart failure, aim for:

*'Doctors should arrange for people with suspected heart failure to be offered appropriate investigations (e.g. electrocardiography, echocardiography) that will confirm or refute the diagnosis. For those individuals in whom heart failure is confirmed its cause should be identified—the treatments most likely to both relieve symptoms and reduce their risk of death should be offered.'*

*Department of Health (2000)*

The Framework made clear that heart failure should be proactively managed and recommended the following as be part of the planned management of care for patients:

- Holistic patient assessment, including risk factors, signs and symptoms
- Relevant investigations, which should include electrocardiography, echocardiography and biochemistry

- Echocardiography should be carried out by a trained operator to include competent interpretation of the result. This could be activated by referral to a specialist heart failure clinic, to cardiology outpatients, or directly to echocardiography from primary care
- Lifestyle advice
- Medical and/or nursing treatment
- Patient education
- Family support
- Regular follow-up and review of the patient and care package and his/her ongoing needs.

This initiative will require clear communication pathways between all professionals concerned and the document goes on to suggest that teams involved in the care of patients with heart failure should meet regularly to discuss clinical issues. It will also include those professionals working in palliative care as the disease progresses and patients and carers face the inevitable process of death and dying.

## The role of the heart failure specialist nurse

Based on heart failure-specific patterns of hospital activity, Stewart et al (2002) undertook research which estimated that the cost of hospital admissions to the NHS was calculated at £166.2 million. They suggested that a home-based programme of specialist nurse management could reduce recurrent bed use by 50% or more, with a resulting annual saving equivalent to £169 000 per 1000 patients treated. The heart failure nurse needs to be experienced in cardiac care, and have an ability to work independently in order to take on responsibilities such as patient assessment, prescribing, and drug titration. People with heart failure need education in order to adapt to their condition, and be supported in self-caring to prevent and reduce hospital admissions. Patient education is an increasingly important component in the management of patients with heart failure and nurses are becoming more involved in this specialist area of clinical work.

There are a range of topics where the heart failure specialist nurse may inform and support the patient:

*General advice relating to heart failure*
- Explain and explore the condition and the prognosis
- Monitoring of symptoms
- Encouraging self-management of symptoms
- Rationale and adherence to treatment

*Physical aspects*
- Daily physical activities rest and exercise
- Work
- Sexual activity

*Lifestyle*
- Restrictions in sodium intake if required
- Restrictions in fluid intake in severe heart failure
- Regulating alcohol intake to within Government guidelines (men 3–4 units per day, women 2–3 units per day) or encouraging abstention
- Smoking cessation
- Weight monitoring and a healthy diet to reduce obesity
- Travel and air flight. Will oxygen be required for the journey? Travel insurance and whether a doctor's certificate of fitness to travel may be required. Consider the risks of developing deep vein thrombosis and peripheral oedema
- Hot and humid conditions may cause fluid loss from sweating and mean a review of diuretic medication

*Medication advice*
- Drug administration
- Adverse drug effects, or signs of intoxication
- Drug interaction and drugs to avoid or be aware of (e.g. non-steroidal anti-inflammatory drugs)
- Flexible diuretic intake

*Health*
- Taking advantage of pneumococcal and influenza immunizations to reduce the risk of developing those infections and putting further strain on the heart
- Concomitant illnesses and infections.

---

**Reflection**

Think about the advice you might give a patient with chronic heart failure to ensure they are compliant with their diuretic therapy.

---

# Living with heart failure

As with any long-term condition, the patient with heart failure will have to adapt to many changes in both lifestyle and approaches to activity, as well as reconsidering their expectations for life and end of life.

## Psychological problems

Individuals with heart failure often acknowledge a multitude of negative feelings about their condition and the effect that it has on their lives. The prospect of an uncertain future, knowing that they have a condition which is incurable and not knowing how long they will live can often cause worry and depression. As previously identified, loss of memory is a common symptom and this can lead to confusion. However, the patient will usually have insight into his/her disordered thought processes and this frequently triggers anxiety, which may in turn cause him/her to become irritable and critical of carers who are trying to help by performing household tasks that the patient used to do him/herself, but is now unable. This may manifest in feelings of guilt at being unable to help with household chores and being dependent on others. Patients may also be resentful at the loss of activities and hobbies that had they had previously enjoyed. In addition to coming to terms with the diagnosis of heart failure, individuals and their families also have to face the prospect that they have a life-limiting illness. They must, therefore, reflect on their prospects and future, and have many decisions and adjustments to make with regard to both lifestyle and relationships. They may go through varying stages of grief before coming to terms with the inevitability of this outcome.

## Adapting activities of living

Many patients feel frustration at no longer being able to do what they used to before developing heart failure, but often they are not given any specific advice about just how much activity it is safe for them to do. Indeed, they may forget the advice they are given because of poor memory, or misunderstand the information that they receive from health professionals. This may cause them to limit their range of activities of living themselves in an attempt to reduce potential hospital admissions, or try to avoid a worsening of their symptoms. As a result, some patients and their carers can become reluctant to leave the home in an attempt to cope with the impact of the disease. This causes both the patient and the carers to become isolated, subsequently affecting their psychological health.

As the heart failure deteriorates, many individuals will also require adaptions to the home in order to maintain their activities of living. There are many aids to living to facilitate self-care and help with washing or dressing for example, but most individuals will require some assistance from a health professional in order to explore those most appropriate for their needs, and will certainly need referring to social services for a home assessment from an occupational therapist. They may require equipment to enable the health professional to assist with care at home, such as a hoist or hospital bed, which can intrude into their personal lives, and cause distress and changes in relationships. In addition, although there are benefits and allowances which can be claimed to help with paying for the extra care required, these can be complex to understand and difficult to obtain. The impact of accepting adaptions to the home can have a profound effect on both the individual and his/her carer. For example, having to move into a downstairs room as a result of reduced mobility may affect the ability of a couple to have an intimate relationship, and may also limit the availability of accommodation to entertain friends and visitors. This will affect the individual from both psychological and social perspectives.

## Dealing with symptoms

The extent to which symptoms impact on quality of life will depend on the stage of heart failure as previously identified in *Table 3.3*. The ability to self-manage the disease therapies and the patient's knowledge base about their treatments will affect the ability to deal with problems as and when they occur, to avoid acute exacerbations occurring, which may result in a hospital admission. Patients may misunderstand the cause of their heart failure or lack knowledge about how to prevent worsening of symptoms, for example by controlling fluid and salt intake, and weighing themselves to check for fluid retention. Some patients are better able to cope than others. Some younger, less symptomatic patients may achieve what they feel to be a good quality of life. Similarly, some older patients, who have preconceptions about ageing, and who may already expect to be able to do less as they get older, may therefore have fewer psychological problems adapting to the limitations that heart failure imposes. Managing the disease will therefore often require support from a range of professionals, which varies in intensity with the pattern of occurrence of symptoms, and the availability and content of this support will affect how well the patient deals with symptoms.

One of the problems which may affect the patient's ability to manage is the unpredictability of symptom occurrence, resulting in days when the patient feels he/she can cope, and others when he/she feels more restricted by the condition. This unpredictability may produce feelings of frustration and defeatism, which may result in patients 'giving up' on self-caring and becoming totally dependent on carer and professional support. It can cause difficulties and anxiety to both patients and their carers, trying to plan day-to-day activities of living around these variations. It may also mean that it raises concerns about why things are happening or appearing to get worse, and this can bring about feelings of helplessness and hopelessness.

Breathlessness is an example of a symptom which will affect the oxygen uptake and lead to feelings of lethargy. An increase in breathlessness may result in an individual not being able to perform activities such as walking, washing or dressing themselves, which on good days they are able to do unaided. Breathlessness at night may also affect sleeping, which will lead to increased feelings of exhaustion and inability to perform activities during the daytime. There may be lack of appetite leading to malnutrition, as the individual cannot face the act of preparing meals, or even eating a large meal, quite apart from whether they are able to shop for food themselves. This is in addition to the symptom of nausea, which is often present and detracts from the enjoyment of eating.

## Coping with other conditions

Patients with heart failure usually have associated underlying diseases and it has been suggested that the risk of hospitalization strongly increases with the number of chronic conditions present (Braunstein et al, 2003). These can include problems such as anaemia, renal disease, and hypertension. Non-cardiac comorbidities such as diabetes or arthritis are also prevalent in older patients with chronic heart failure, and are frequently associated with adverse clinical outcomes. This seems almost inevitable when you consider the implications. Managing activities of living when you are both breathless and also less mobile or dextrous becomes an almost impossible hurdle to face. Choosing a meal which will fit into your diabetic diet may become an ordeal when you are exhausted by the effort of food preparation. Depression may lead to state of apathy about testing blood sugars, or self-medicating with insulin or tablets. Memory-loss may mean that forgetting to take insulin medication at the correct times. At this stage, the impact that heart failure has on diabetes will seriously affect the individual's health and wellbeing, with disastrous results on the clinical outcomes.

## Difficulties with managing multiple medications

Patients with heart failure will require medication regimens to improve and maintain circulation, as well as to control other symptoms occurring as a result of heart failure. The side-effects of medications frequently cause difficulties and many patients have suggested that they sometimes feel that some medications were not useful, but were actually making them feel more unwell, caused by some side-effects such as hypotension and gastrointestinal upsets. Patients may require a combination of drugs, all to be taken at different times of the day, and either before or after meals in a regimen which needs to be carefully managed, and this can take over his/her life. Many individuals report an increasing inability to remember things as their heart failure develops (Vogels et al, 2007). As a result, there will be increased anxiety about managing the sometimes complex drug regimens required, especially if there is comorbidity—the presence of other diseases requiring treatments such as arthritis, which often occurs in the elderly. Trying to remember to keep hospital and clinic appointments where medication is often reviewed may also become problematic, and remembering the medicating advice they had been given at these appointments becomes difficult and concerning.

## Changing roles and relationships within the family

Changes in the patient's role within the family and a loss of social relationships are common problems, and having to rely on others causes a great deal of concern both to patients and their carers. In younger individuals where an inability to continue to work occurs, worries about finances may be an issue. Loss of role within the family unit as a wage earner may compound the feelings of frustration and sense of worthlessness. It may also lead to another burden being placed on the partner, who may be forced to give up work in order to become the main carer. These changes can lead to reduced income within the household and impact on levels of deprivation. Such levels of poverty are often made worse if a patient's ability to manage to live a normal life is a result of the disease, especially if he/she requires environmental adaptations such as a stair lift or bathing aids, but is not able to afford them. Difficulties in accessing benefits such as income support, disability allowance, or social services assessments, can be complex procedures and crammed with bureaucracy and form-filling, and often make individuals feel degraded, causing great distress for some.

## Cultural and religious issues

These problems are particularly acute for those with language differences and who may have a lack of knowledge of how to access the health and social care services for the support needed. In the UK, the availability of an interpreter is essential for all non-English speaking patients and their families accessing the NHS, in order that they fully understand heart failure and its treatment. In addition, language difficulties can restrict opportunities for support delivered by telephone, which limits the availability of the information that some may receive. The introduction of telemedicine will be particularly problematic in these situations. There are noticeable cultural differences in the way some ethnic minority groups may consider the implications of heart failure in relation to the meaning of their condition and beliefs about the effects of treatment. They may consult a traditional healer rather than access the services of the NHS. Believers in Allah may feel supported by their cultural philosophy of the inevitability of their situation and derive comfort from prayer and spiritual beliefs, especially those concerning dying and death. The discipline and practice of Islam in relation to knowledge and understanding about diet, exercise and general health may provide reassurance to some. On a more negative note, the difficulties surrounding ritual ablutions—not being able to wash before daily prayers, and not being able to kneel or prostrate during prayers—may cause some individuals to feel troubled and guilty, and increase feelings of depression.

---

**Reflection**

- Patients with chronic heart failure often have negative feelings about their long-term health
- With reference to this statement, consider measures that may be implemented by the multidisciplinary team to promote the patient's psychosocial wellbeing.

---

# The future

The population aged 65 years and over is expected to rise dramatically over the next 30 years. As the population becomes increasingly elderly, and since the elderly are more susceptible to the development of heart failure, it is likely that there may be increasing numbers of people in the population who will suffer from heart failure. The role of GPs in accurate diagnosis and of specialist nurses in effective management of people with heart failure is key to reducing hospital admissions for the condition. Government guidelines are aimed at relieving symptoms, slowing progression of the condition, and maximizing quality of life (DH, 2003). This can be achieved by drug, non-drug and surgical approaches. With the exception of surgery, much of this management can be carried out within the primary care setting. Although treatments such as heart transplants are now much more common than 20 years ago, the availability of donor organs may become more of a problem as the donating population also ages. Other more conservative treatments are being developed with the creation of new and more effective medication agents. However, the only certain way to minimize the condition will be a proactive approach to assess high-risk groups within the population and modify the behaviour and lifestyle of susceptible groups.

Braunstein JB, Anderson GF, Gerstenblith G et al (2003) Noncardiac comorbidity increases preventable hospitalizations and mortality among Medicare beneficiaries with chronic heart failure. *J Am Coll Cardiol* **42**(7): 1226–33

British Heart Foundation (2006) Mortality from heart failure. http://tinyurl.com/yhuhn57 (accessed 27 October 2009)

Cowie MR, Wood DA, Coats AJ et al (2000) Survival of patients with a new diagnosis of heart failure: a population-based study. *Heart* **83**(5): 505–10

Cowie MR (2001) The prognosis of heart failure: the view from the real world. *Eur Heart J* **22**(15): 1247–8

DH (2000) *National Service Framework for Coronary Heart Disease*. Department of Health, London. ref: 2000

DH (2003) *Developing services for heart failure*. DH, London. ref: 2003

Healthcare Commission (2007) Pushing the boundaries: Improving the series for people with heart failure. http://tinyurl.com/yaqjs5n (accessed 8 October 2009)

Hunt L (2008) How to close the readmission revolving door. http://tinyurl.com/yls4473 (accessed 27 October 2009)

Joint Formulary Committee (2009) *British National Formulary* 58. September. BMJ Publishing Group Ltd and RPS Publishing, London

Peattie P.I, Walker S (1995) *Understanding Nursing Care*. Churchill Livingstone, Edinburgh

Raphael C, Briscoe C, Davies J et al (2007) Limitations of the New York Heart Association functional classification system and self-reported walking distances in chronic heart failure. *Heart* **93**(4): 476–82

Stewart S, Blue L, Walker A, Morrison C, McMurray JJ (2002) An economic analysis of specialist heart failure nurse management in the UK; can we afford not to implement it? *Eur Heart J* **23**(17): 1369–78

The King's Fund (2009) Predicting and Reducing Re-admission to Hospital. http://tinyurl.com/ya9pzc5 (accessed 27 October 2009)

Vogels RL, Scheltens P, Schroeder-Tanka JM, Weinstein HC (2007) Cognitive impairment in heart failure: a systematic review of the literature. *Eur J Heart Fail* **9**(5): 440–9

Wood DA (2002) Preventing clinical heart failure: the rationale and scientific evidence. *Heart* **88**(Suppl 2): ii15–22

# CHAPTER 4

# Stroke

*Cheryl Utecht*

Stroke is characterized by an acute loss of focal brain function lasting more than 24 hours or leading to death, which is thought to be the result of spontaneous haemorrhage or inadequate blood supply to a part of the brain as a result of low blood flow, thrombosis or embolism, associated with diseases of the blood vessels, heart or blood (Warlow et al, 2000). Reading this chapter and reflecting on your own experiences should enable you to achieve the following learning outcomes:

- To understand the impact of stroke on lifestyle and quality of life
- To understand the role of the multidisciplinary team in the prevention and management of stroke
- To consider ways of supporting patients with ongoing management following a stroke.

## Background

Each year in the UK, 110 000 people suffer a first stroke, and approximately 25% of these people will be under 65 years old. In England, stroke is the third largest cause of disability, which results in approximately 300 000 people living with a severe or moderate disability. The cost of stroke to the NHS and the economy is £7 billion per year in direct costs (Department of Health [DH], 2007).

Over the past 10 years, there have been a number of policies and guidelines published to enhance the evidence-based care of stroke patients, including the Royal College of Physicians' (RCP) *National Clinical Guidelines* (2004), the *National Service Framework* [NSF] *for Older People* (DH, 2001), and more recently, the *National Stroke Strategy* (DH, 2007).

Stroke is a condition that aligns with the *NSF for Long-Term Conditions* (DH, 2005a) owing to the complexity of disability sustained. This NSF recommends that a structured and systematic approach is key to improving the care of individuals with a long-term condition (DH, 2005a). The model uses a tiered approach, which recognizes that levels of intervention depend on the degree of need relating to effectively supporting those with a long-term condition. The focus is on health promotion, self-care and support, disease management, and complex case management. This chapter uses this framework to explore and discuss each level of need and how it relates to the management of the stroke patient.

## Health promotion

The *National Stroke Strategy* (DH, 2007) has highlighted the need to raise awareness of the risk factors and signs of stroke (*Table 4.1*). Promoting healthy living is an important aspect of stroke prevention, especially in those who are economically disadvantaged as they are more likely to be at a higher risk of stroke. Similarly, people of African–Caribbean and South Asian origin are at a higher risk of stroke, and therefore health promotion is an important aspect to consider for these groups (DH, 2007).

Health promotion activities that could reduce the risk of stroke should be developed within the primary care setting; these include smoking cessation, and monitoring for hypertension and irregular heartbeats. Although there have been no randomized controlled trials, it has been suggested that stroke can be decreased by at least 1.5-times by implementing such strategies (Hankey, 2004).

The Government's recent initiative, *Putting prevention first* (DH, 2008a), involves a health check for people over 45 years, examining their risk of heart disease, hypertension, stroke and diabetes. It is envisaged that

---

### Table 4.1 Main risk factors for stroke

- Increasing age
- Hypertension
- Diabetes
- Ethnic group
- Family history
- Previous stroke or transient ischaemic attack (TIA)
- Ischaemic heart disease
- Smoking
- Obesity
- Excessive alcohol consumption
- Sedentary lifestyle

the practice nurse may have a significant role in this initiative; however, it can be combined with other health professionals, for example the pharmacist can offer cholesterol checks and advice on smoking cessation.

The *National Stroke Strategy* indicates that by using health promotion programmes, approximately 20 000 strokes could be prevented every year (DH, 2007). These programmes can be implemented in primary care trusts (PCTs), with GPs managing the risk factors according to national guidelines, for example (RCP, 2004). The voluntary sector could also provide a range of health promotion schemes, for example the Stroke Association has such a programme in Hull, which helps individuals identify lifestyle changes to reduce the risk of stroke or recurrent stroke. Other ideas for healthy living could be the referral of patients to exercise classes and weight management programmes.

Improved health promotion has the potential to reduce the risk of stroke, but of equal importance is raising the individuals' knowledge to recognize the signs and symptoms of stroke once it starts. Prompt medical attention can be beneficial in reducing the risk of disability and increasing the chance of a good recovery (NHS Choices, 2009). Rapid diagnosis is important to identify the cause of the stroke, assess the level of damage, and for an early start to appropriate treatment. The *National Stroke Strategy* (DH, 2007) recommends an early brain scan to determine the cause, severity and area of the brain affected. It is equally important to appreciate that early recognition and emergency action is also considered necessary in the event of a transient ischaemic attack (TIA). The signs and symptoms of a TIA are the same as those for stroke, but a TIA is defined as 'a clinical syndrome characterized by the acute loss of focal brain function lasting less than 24 hours (Hankey, 2004). A TIA may be indistinguishable in the early stages from a full stroke. The DH's (2009) awareness programme 'Act F.A.S.T.' (Face, Arm, Speech, Time test) is aimed to educate both the public and professionals in the early recognition and response to the signs of a stroke or TIA.

For those who have previously had a stroke or TIA, health education is even more important. Patients should be assessed for risk factors and given information about lifestyle modification to reduce the risk of a further stroke. These patients should be referred to a specialist clinic where they can be assessed and appropriate treatments accessed (RCP, 2004). It may also be advisable to provide patients with information relating to voluntary organizations for psychological and social support, such as the Stroke Association.

For patients who have suffered a first stroke, there is a need for health professionals to provide education as secondary prevention, and this may include some of the activities already mentioned. Allied health professionals may address specific aspects of care. For example, the physiotherapist may offer advice with regard to the correct positioning of limbs to prevent deformity or spasticity. The speech and language therapist will focus on the maintenance of the swallow reflex and the correct type of diet.

---

### Case study

*John is a 49-year-old lorry driver who has suffered a transient ischaemic attack (TIA). He is clinically obese, takes little exercise, and smokes 30 cigarettes every day. John has little understanding of what a TIA is or how this could affect his occupation.*

- Consider what advice you may give to this patient
- What agencies might you involve in this aspect of care?
- What obstacles could there be in John obtaining health promotion advice?

---

## Self care/support

The *National Stroke Strategy* aim for life after stroke is for patients, relatives and carers, whether in care homes or at home, to achieve a good quality of life and maximize independence, wellbeing and choice (DH, 2007). The support needed by stroke patients has a commonality with those living with a long-term condition, and therefore, the *NSF for Long-Term Conditions* (DH, 2005a) and *NSF for Older People* (DH, 2001) are of significant relevance.

For most people with a long-term condition, diagnosis often follows a period of uncertainty in which the individual may have experienced a range of signs and symptoms, which following consultation, examination and investigation, result in a definitive diagnosis. This allows the individual in some part to come to terms with the implications and resultant adaption and life changes their diagnosis may bring. However, for the individual who suffers a stroke, the experience is all too often sudden and unexpected. The rapid onset and devastating effects of resultant disability, coupled with the knowledge that they have suffered a stroke, often leaves the patient feeling vulnerable and unable to cope with the unexpected onset of a potentially life-threatening long-term condition.

Given the correct level of support, 70–80% of people can live with and manage their condition (DH, 2005b). To be able to do this, nurses and allied health professionals need to provide education and support to enable the patient to care for him/herself. *Supporting People with Long-Term Conditions*

(DH, 2005b) describes the nurse and allied health professional as facilitators in directing the patient and carer to the appropriate resource or person. This enables the patient to be aware of the options available to them. Examples of this could be the use of assisted technology that can help support self-care or providing appropriate information regarding stroke support and carers groups. Many patients are discharged home following a stroke with some disability and will need to access services within the community, for both physical and psychological support.

Physical disability is the most obvious effect of stroke, and there is support and help available to patients in the community to continue with the rehabilitation process. In recent years, a number of schemes have been introduced to provide care at or closer to home. The Government, in *Our health, Our care, Our say* (DH, 2006), discusses the need to provide the right level of support. Some of the aspects addressed are choice and control, personal dignity, and improved quality of life. For some stroke patients having to manage with a mild to moderate disability, there may be issues relating to dignity, for example the need to have carers in to provide personal care in the home environment. Some people may find this difficult to accept when they have previously been independent. Providing such support, however, can lead to the patient having control and choice to improve his/her quality of life.

For this group of patients, there should be a tailored, flexible approach to rehabilitation—some patients may still be of working age and want to return to their job. For this reason, there needs to be a coordinated partnership between professionals, not just in health and social care, but including housing departments, employment advisors, and leisure and transport facilities.

Psychological support is an aspect of stroke care that is sometimes not as high profile as addressing physical disability. It has been identified that most stroke patients have feelings of loss and grieve for the past 'self' (Thompson, 2008). These patients, therefore, do need psychological support as they have or are going through a bereavement process—they are now seen as disabled or see themselves as disabled. In younger patients this may be relevant with regard to their role in society. These patients may have to consider a change of job, or even leave employment with their partner becoming the 'breadwinner'. It is important to consider this as it may lead the patient to lose his/her identity and role in the partnership/family, and can lead to feelings of helplessness and frustration on both sides (Thompson, 2008). Psychological support should also consider coping strategies, emotional issues, sexuality and sexual function. Sexuality and sexual function post-stroke is often neglected by health professionals owing to its sensitivity and being considered a private matter. This should, however, be discussed and the patient can then be offered appropriate advice through the relevant agencies, and counselling if necessary.

> **Case study**
>
> Nila is 52 years old and has suffered a right-sided stroke, which has left her with a left hemiplegia and dysphasia. Nila needs some help with washing and dressing, but she is quite determined to go home and continue with her rehabilitation in her own surroundings. The family is supportive of this, but have concerns about how she will manage when they are at work. As a result of her dysphasia, Nila has been reluctant to try and talk as she feels embarrassed.
>
> * What support could be offered to Nila and her family in the form of voluntary agencies?
> * Consider what rehabilitation services would be available to a patient like Nila in your area
> * How can Nila be encouraged to express herself?

## Disease and care management

Some patients will require a more active approach. They are those who are at risk of complications from their condition and will therefore benefit from the services of the multidisciplinary team. GPs and specialist nurses can make a significant contribution by assisting the patient to manage his/her condition in a proactive manner and avoid future complications.

If disease management is proactive it can make a real difference to stroke patients who may experience a range of problems, which may threaten their health and wellbeing. The NSFs (DH, 2001; 2005) have already demonstrated that this approach can have a significant impact on the outcomes for these patients. By using a disease management approach, the health professional can ensure better management, reduce disability, and produce better health outcomes.

For people who have suffered a stroke, there is a need to acknowledge that this can occur again. Secondary prevention is therefore an important aspect of disease management. This relies on the members of the multidisciplinary team ensuring that the patient is managed in a proactive manner.

The stroke physician will consider what medication, if any, is appropriate for the patient. There are a number of regimens that may be considered and this will depend on the type of stroke and risk factors. In association with this, all GPs must now have a register of patients who have experienced a stroke, which should enable the seamless transfer from the hospital to community setting. The *National Stroke Strategy* (DH, 2007) recognizes that the provision of a link between inpatient and community care is vital for effective long-term care. The Darzi Report (DH, 2008b) indicates that this may be undertaken by agreeing care plans with the patient and having a named professional to organize services for the needs of the patient.

The *NSF for Long-Term Conditions* (2005a) argues that the patient's needs should be identified early and that the response to these needs is prompt to address the appropriate care or support. Patients post-stroke are at risk of complications from their condition. It is this group of patients which benefits from the intervention of the multidisciplinary team.

Nurses in general practice and specialist nurses have a key contribution to make in the support of these people, by being proactive in helping the patient to manage his/her condition and avoid complications. Nurses are ideally placed to build a relationship with the patient and his/her family. The Royal College of Nursing (RCN) (2000) framework for the rehabilitation nurse is an example of how the nurse's role can be central to the rehabilitation of patients. It suggests that nurses are in a unique position to gather information and make good use of contact time in a therapeutic manner. For nurses, this may be using a variety of communication skills and actively listening to the patient's concerns. The nurse can be the co-coordinator for the rest of the multidisciplinary team, and is often a first point of contact.

Other health professionals have an important role to play with this group of patients to prevent complications and reduce readmissions. Physiotherapists are often the prominent focus for the stroke patient. In dealing with care management, the physiotherapist is in a strong position to provide treatment, give advice, and could be the co-coordinator for the patient's care plan.

The occupational therapist may assess for adaptions to the home and provide support in the early stages post-discharge as part of an intermediate care team with other professionals. Providing advice on how to dress, for example, using aids or different techniques can promote independence and raise self-esteem.

Some stroke patients may require the services of a speech and language therapist. Patients who have some form of dysphasia may find it difficult to get back into society for fear of embarrassment. The other aspect of care for the speech and language therapist is dysphagia, which may require a special diet.

For patients who are care-managed, there need to be clear lines of communication between different services and the multidisciplinary team to enable the patient to have some control over his/her condition. The other aspect to being able to manage their condition is to have contact with voluntary agencies who may provide peer support, advice and guidance. This group of patients may have some significant disability, but this can be managed effectively if a good assessment and care plan have been agreed by all members of the team and the patient.

There is now the recognition that the patient should be encouraged to take responsibility for his/her own care (DH, 2005a). This role has been developed as the Expert Patients Programme (DH, 2007), which highlights the ability of the patient to become an 'expert' and values the knowledge that patients acquire about his/her condition or disease. Expert patients are described as being in control and confident, effective at communicating with professionals and willing to share responsibility, realistic about the impact of their condition on themselves and their family, and use their skills and knowledge to enhance their quality of life. This is particularly important for younger stroke patients who have the prospect of many years in front of them, in which they have to consider family, employment and financial matters.

Finally, an important aspect of care management is the promotion of health. All stroke patients should be advised of the need to manage their lifestyle through diet, smoking habits, levels of exercise, and alcohol intake. The nurse has a valuable role to play by providing ongoing support and education, making any necessary referrals, and directing patients to other agencies and services for ongoing support or advice.

Stroke is a condition that can involve a number of professionals from the multidisciplinary team. The essence at this level of care is communication to enable a seamless journey. The journey begins before discharge, with patients and carers involved in arrangements and organization. Stroke patients and their carers value continuity, which includes being kept informed and having a clear and constant point of contact with services. The aim for this group of patients should be to plan for tailored and flexible rehabilitation, which will affect their long-term recovery and reduce long-term disability.

---

### Case study

*Mr Martin is a 60-year-old, retired sales representative who has suffer a right-sided stroke. He has a left hemiplegia, but is now managing to walk a short distance with a stick. Mr Martin does have mild dysphagia and is taking a soft diet. He lives with his wife, and before the stroke enjoyed going to the pub and socializing with friends.*

* Who would be the significant members of the multidisciplinary team involved in the care of Mr Martin?
* Where may you advise Mr Martin to seek help?
* Consider how Mr Martin may be able to manage his condition and continue to live a fulfilled life.

---

# Patients with complex conditions

The final group of patients are those with complex issues. These patients are those with a higher risk of unplanned hospital admissions or long-term institutionalization, and can be identified as those who have a degenerative disease with one or two more chronic conditions (DH, 2005b). This may involve the patient taking several different medications or having problems with the activities of daily living. To manage these patients, the *NSF for Long-Term Conditions* (DH, 2005a) advocates the use of case management. Nurses known as community matrons are responsible for managing these patients and have an active caseload of approximately 50 patients with highly complex needs. The nurse is able to perform a high-level assessment to help patients negotiate not only the health and social care systems, but also involve other agencies, for example those dealing with housing, transport, education, and employment. This is especially important for stroke patients who may have other existing conditions. As previously mentioned, stroke patients are often seen by several members of the multidisciplinary team and for complex cases, it is essential that there are clear lines of communication. The role of the community matron is to enable the patient to make personal choices about their care, which may include the decision to stay at home until the end of life.

This care then involves both the physical and psychosocial aspects of the patient's life. Physically, some patients can be severely disabled and therefore a number of issues should be considered and discussed with the patient and his/her family. This should begin before discharge from hospital to ensure a seamless journey. Some of the issues to consider are outlined below.

### Who is going to be the main carer? is it going to be the partner, a relative, or a care agency?

Not all patients would want their partner or relative to provide intimate personal care for them. Equally, the partner may not wish to do this either. It is essential that this discussion takes place before discharge and arrangements organized. As the older population increases, there is the possibility that the person who has suffered a stroke could have previously been the main carer for his/her partner. This situation then puts increased physical and psychological pressure on the family as to how to cope with these demands. As health professionals, this is a situation that is becoming more common and there is a need to work collaboratively with other agencies to achieve the best for these patients, whether they remain at home or need to enter sheltered or residential care.

## Suitable accommodation

People who have had a severe stroke may find that their accommodation is now no longer suitable. There may be several solutions to this, for example simple pieces of equipment, stair rails, and raised toilet seats. Other issues may be to facilitate access, through the building of ramps, widening doorways for wheelchair access, and integrating stair lifts, all of which are available through local councils and grants. Most of the physical aspects can be addressed with forms of adaption, the provision of equipment and the use of care agencies

Psychosocial aspects of stroke are not as easy to address and can be devastating to some patients, therefore having a central person to contact can be beneficial for both the patient and the family.

## Emotional difficulties

Many people experience emotional difficulties following a stroke. This can have an impact on their long-term physical rehabilitation. Emotional problems can lead to depression and isolation. Mauk (2006) describes the psychological aspect of the post-stroke journey as having a variety of phases. This begins with 'agonizing', where the patient and family are interested only in the physical aspects of progression and there is a general sense of doom and loss. As recovery progresses, the patient experiences a variety of differing emotions, which leads to the second stage of 'fantasizing'; feeling a sense of loss and 'unreality'. The 'realizing' phase is when the patient begins to accept and acknowledge the problems resulting from the stroke. The enormity of the event does become more apparent and patients have identified this as a 'culture shock'. As the patient's rehabilitation continues, he/she begins to 'blend', or start trying to move on and aspire to normality. The final two phases of the journey are 'framing', in which the patient starts making sense of his/her life; and 'owning', which is the last stage of post-stroke adaption, where the survivor begins to take responsibility and control over his/her own health.

During this period, it would seem appropriate that the patient has a 'case manager/matron' as a central figure from which to seek advice and support. The nurse can help the patient through the transition, exploring areas that concern the patient and by trying to establish any interests he/she may have. It is important to remember that during this time the carer may also need psychological support in coming to terms with their partner's condition. Part of the nurse's role would be to offer psychological support themselves, or refer to other allied health professionals involved in the delivery of psychological care. Voluntary organizations can offer local stroke clubs, which may provide peer support for these patients. For carers, there are also local and national carer agencies providing counselling and sitting services.

### Younger stroke patients

This group of patients a number of have different needs. They may have a family to support and issues surrounding employment. It is not always easy to find peer support groups for these patients, as most stroke clubs are geared towards the older person. The nurse needs to be aware of the complexity of this small group of patients and can be the facilitator for referring to other agencies, for example a disability advisor at the employment and family support agencies.

The role of the nurse in these complex cases is pivotal as they act as co-coordinator in most cases of the multidisciplinary team. The role provides the patient with a central figure they can communicate with, rather than not knowing who is responsible for their care. This also helps in preventing none-essential readmissions to hospital as most problems may be able to be managed in the community setting, which is beneficial for both patients and their families.

---

### Case study

*Sidney is a 72-year-old African–Caribbean man who has suffered a left-sided stroke, which has resulted in a severe right-sided hemiplegia, dysphagia, and loss of sensation to the lips and mouth. Sidney has atrial fibrillation, for which he takes warfarin and also has diabetes, which is managed by oral medication. Discharge has been discussed and Sidney is adamant that he wants to go home. Sidney's wife is finding it difficult to cope as she suffers from arthritis and is suffering increased pain, which means she cannot cope with her duties as a carer.*

* Consider the role of the community matron
* What services may be available in your area for Sidney?
* How would it be possible for Sidney to remain at home?
* Consider what help may be available for Sidney's wife.

# Conclusion

This chapter has addressed stroke care using the framework detailed in *Supporting People with Long-Term Conditions* (DH, 2005b). The framework identifies that the majority of patients can have control over their condition, but recognizes that there are different levels of need moving from self-care to more complex conditions and problems. The *National Stroke Strategy* (DH, 2007) and the *NSF for Long-Term Conditions* (DH, 2005) are useful tools to guide the health professional in the care and management of the stroke patient. The discussion provides the reader with some pointers and scenarios that can be used in the discussion and care of stroke patients.

DH (2001) *National Service Framework for Older People*. DH, London: ref 2001

DH (2004) General Medical Services Contract. http://tinyurl.com/yjccfgt (accessed 13 October 2009)

DH (2005a) *National Service Framework for Long-Term Conditions*. DH, London: ref 2005

DH (2005b) *Supporting People with Long-Term Conditions: Liberating the talents of nurses who care for people with long term conditions*. DH, London: ref 3853

DH (2006) Our health, Our care, Our say. http://tinyurl.com/yvkmdx (accessed 13 October 2009)

DH (2007) National Stroke Strategy. DH, London: ref 9025

DH (2008a) *Putting Prevention First*. DH, London

DH (2008b) *High Quality Care for All: NHS Next Stage Review final report*. DH, London: ref 10106

DH (2009) Stroke: Act F.A.S.T. awareness campaign. http://tinyurl.com/cpnoo6 (accessed 13 October 2009)

Hankey GJ (2004) *Stroke: Your Questions Answered*. Churchill Livingstone, London

Mauk KL (2006) Nursing interventions within the Mauk model of Poststroke Recovery. *Rehabil Nurs* **31**(6): 257–63

NHS Choices (2009) Understanding stroke and TIA. http://tinyurl.com/ygnv24r (accessed 13 October 2009)

Royal College of Nursing (2000) *Role of the Rehabilitation Nurse*. RCN publications, London

Royal College of Physicians (2004) *National Clinical Guidelines for Stroke*. 2nd edn. Royal College of Physicians, London

Thompson H (2008) A review of the psychosocial consequences of stroke and their impact on spousal relationships. *Br J Neurosci Nurs* **4**(4) 117–84

Warlow CP, Dennis MS, van Gijn J et al (2000) *Stroke: a practical guide to management.* Oxford Blackwell Scientific Publications, UK

## Useful websites

*The Stroke Association: www.stroke.org.uk*
*Different Strokes: www.differentstrokes.co.uk*

# CHAPTER 5

# Chronic obstructive pulmonary disease

*Ron Eldridge*

The National Institute for Health and Clinical Excellence (NICE) define chronic obstructive pulmonary disease (COPD) as:

> *'COPD is characterised by airflow obstruction. The airflow obstruction is usually progressive, not fully reversible and does not change markedly over several months. The disease is predominantly caused by smoking.'*
> *National Institute for Health and Clinical Excellence (2004)*

This chapter explores the long-term conditions grouped under the heading of COPD. The aim is to provide an understanding of some of the problems and issues which may affect the life and experiences of the individual with a diagnosis of COPD. Reading this chapter and reflecting on your own experiences should enable you to achieve the following learning outcomes:

*   Review your knowledge and understanding of COPD
*   Understand the impact COPD has on lifestyle and quality of life
*   An awareness of the impact smoking has on the development of COPD
*   An understanding of holistic assessment of an individual with COPD
*   Examine the management strategies enabling individuals to manage the effects of COPD.

## Background

COPD is a very broad diagnosis with conditions being grouped into two clinical subtypes. Patients with emphysema are sometimes referred to as 'blue bloaters', owing to the often blue complexion (cyanosis). In this condition, damage to lung tissue and the small air sacs (the alveoli at the end of the airways) causes air to become trapped in the lungs, leading to shortness of breath. The other subtype is chronic bronchitis, in which inflammation occurs in the bronchial tubes, causing narrowing of the airways and making breathing difficult. These patients may not appear to be cyanosed, and hence may be described as 'pink puffers'. These subtypes may be further classified as being mild, moderate or severe (National Collaborating Centre for Chronic Conditions [NCCCC], 2004). While COPD patients may exhibit signs and symptoms of both conditions, it is important to appreciate that they each have a different pathology (Bourke, 2003).

## Chronic bronchitis

Chronic bronchitis (or type A COPD) typically presents with an inflammation of the bronchi that leads to narrowing and obstruction of the airways. This inflammation stimulates the production of mucus and in turn causes the patient to have a productive cough. The risks of bacterial lung infections are increased with such mucoid obstruction of the airways. Pure chronic bronchitis, however, is clinically defined as an otherwise unexplained chronic productive cough for at least three months in each of two successive years (Bobadilla et al, 2002). A total of 85% of patients with COPD have chronic bronchitis (Barnes, 2000; Global Initiative for Chronic Obstructive Lung Disease [GOLD], 2004). Clinical features may include:

- Daily productive cough for three months to a year or more
- Puffy, hyperventilated breathing with pursed lips on expiration (i.e. pink puffer)
- Pink or reddish complexion (i.e. pink puffer)
- An increased respiratory rate tachypnoea (i.e. pink puffer)
- Frequent exacerbations with no apparent infection
- No polycythaemia (an increase in red blood cells in excess of 6–9 million per cubic millilitre of blood. Causative factors include smoking, lung and heart disease)
- Typically thin or cachectic — a general physical wasting or malnutrition associated with chronic disease
- May develop *cor pulmonale*
- No carbon dioxide ($CO_2$) retention.

## Emphysema

Patients suffering from emphysema (type B COPD) will experience permanent enlargement of the alveoli owing to the destruction of the walls between the alveoli. This reduces the elasticity of the lungs, which in turn leads to the collapse of the bronchioles resulting in restricted airflow from the alveoli. This causes a cycle whereby air is trapped in the damaged alveoli, thus reducing the lungs' ability to deflate during exhalation. This then reduces the lungs' ability to expand sufficiently with the next breath and as a consequence, reduces the amount of air inhaled and the extent to which a sufficient exchange of gasses can take place (Holleman and Simel, 1995; Petty, 2002). The destruction of the alveolar walls also decreases the number of capillaries available for the gaseous exchange. The respiratory process may be compromised further in that the semi-inflated, damaged alveoli may compress adjacent, less damaged lung tissue, preventing it from functioning to its fullest capacity. Clinical features may include:

* Dry cough or no cough
* Prolonged inspiration and expiration of breath
* Wheeze
* Marked cyanosis, especially the lips (i.c. blue bloater)
* Peripheral oedema, usually indicative of right-sided heart failure which might lead to cor pulmonale (i.e. blue bloater)
* Overweight (i.e. blue bloater)
* Recurrent infections
* Distended neck veins
* Secondary polycythaemia.

---

**Reflection**

* Have you nursed a patient with a diagnosis of COPD?
* Did this patient have type A or type B?

---

While COPD is associated with smoking, there are a number of other potential precursors to the development of the condition, including environmental pollutants, occupational-related irritants, and occasionally, genetic conditions, such as occupational related irritants (Minkoff, 2005), anti-protease enzyme deficiency, hypertension and atherogenic dyslipidemia (Vicgi et al, 2001). The condition is characterized by the gradual progression of irreversible airflow obstruction (Dewar and Curry, 2006) and increased inflammation in the airways and lung parenchyma (that is, the key elements essential to the functioning of the lung). At best, the airflow obstruction may be partially reversible with bronchodilator therapy (NCCCC, 2004)

# The anatomy and physiology of breathing

In order to understand the changes that take place in COPD, it is important to have a working knowledge of the anatomy and physiology of the healthy respiratory system to better appreciate the pathology of COPD.

During the act of breathing, air enters the upper respiratory tract, through the mouth and the nostrils (nares), where small hairs (*vibrissae*) filter dust and other debris. The air then enters the nasal passages, the posterior walls of which comprise the conchae, sometimes known as turbinates. The conchae warm and moisten the air before it passes into the nasopharynx. The mucus layer traps finer debris from the inhaled air, which the cilia (small hair-like projections) carry to the pharynx to be swallowed. Air passes from the nasal cavity into the nasopharynx through a pair of posterior openings in the nasal cavity (choanae). The upper respiratory tract then connects to the lower via the oropharynx and the laryngopharynx.

The lower respiratory tract comprises the conducting airways (the trachea, bronchi, and lungs) and *acinus* (the respiratory bronchioles, alveoli, and alveolar sacs). The *acinus* is important as it serves as the area of gas exchange. Within the *acinus*, terminal bronchioles branch into smaller respiratory bronchioles. These feed directly into alveoli at sites along their walls. Lining the lower tract is mucous membrane, which like the conchae contains cilia, and keep the tract clean and move debris up, where it is either swallowed or expectorated.

The alveolar walls contain two basic types of epithelial cells:

- The most plentiful are type I cells. It is across these thin, flat squamous cells that gaseous exchange takes place
- Type II cells provide a vital function in the respiratory process by secreting surfactant. This substance is a lipoprotein, the function of which is to reduce surface tension. This increases pulmonary compliance, allowing the lungs to inflate much more easily, reducing the work involved in breathing, and preventing the lungs from collapsing at the end of expiration.

The reduction in surface tension also reduces the fluid accumulation in the alveolus as surface tension draws fluid across the alveolar wall.

## What goes wrong in COPD?

The increased inflammatory response in the airways in patients with COPD causes mucous glands to enlarge and over-secrete (hypersecretion), resulting in the cilia becoming clogged and knotted with mucus (ciliary dysfunction).

There are also changes to the squamous cells (squamous metaplasia) in the lining of the airways early in the course of the disease (Dewar and Curry, 2006; Puchelle et al, 2006). The ongoing cycle of inflammation and repair results in the thickening and narrowing of the small airways walls, restricting airflow—this is a major mechanism in the increased severity of COPD (Araya et al, 2007). Smokers are often found to have squamous metaplasia, which is an indicator of the body's response to stress and irritation. If the original cells are not robust enough to withstand the new environment in which they find themselves, they change to another type of cell more suited to the new conditions.

As a result of the oxidative irritant damage caused to the pulmonary epithelium, macrophages (also called histiocytes) are stimulated by the inflammation where they defend against invading organisms. Macrophages are efficient phagocytes (cells that ingest microorganisms). When mobilized at an infection site, they phagocytize cellular remains and promote wound healing. COPD patients also have a high neutrophil count, which are the most plentiful of the polymorphonuclear leukocytes and increase dramatically in response to inflammation and infection. Neutrophils are the principal constituent of pus, are highly mobile, and engulf, digest and dispose of invading organisms by phagocytosis. The cytotoxic T-cell (CD8+ T-cells; responsible for lyzing target cells and killing virus infected cells) counts will be raised; these are the smallest of the white blood cells and originate from stem cells in the bone marrow. Cytotoxic T cells directly attack virus infected cells and tumour cells (as opposed to B-lymphocytes, which produce antibodies against specific antigens).

The downside to this response is that the neutrophils and macrophages release inflammatory proteases, elastases and cytokines. A protease is an enzyme that digests proteins by a process of proteolysis, which is the precursor to catabolism, the breakdown of molecules into smaller units resulting in the release of energy. Elastase is also an enzyme from the class of proteases, which break down elastin or elastic fibre, which together with collogen, determine the properties of connective (epithelial) tissue. Cytokines are a type of protein that are vital to the development of the immune response. These use an imbalance of the pro-inflammatory (e.g. environmental pollutants and irritants) and the protective mediators found in the healthy lung (Barnes, 2000; Rennard, 2002).

# The shocking statistics

It is estimated that one sixth of the adult population in the UK smoke— approximately 10 million people, of which 80% began smoking as teenagers

(Action on Smoking and Health [ASH], 2006). Smokers make up to 600 000 visits to the GP every year because of smoking-related conditions (Tobacco Advisory Group, 2000). The cost to the NHS for treating smoking-related diseases is £2.5 billion and growing, an increase of £1 billion in just 10 years (ASH, 2006), even though the NHS has spent £61 million on smoking cessation programmes (NHS Information Centre, 2008)

Approximately 80 000 people die each year in the UK as a result of smoking-related diseases, of which 238 078 deaths are attributable to COPD (Office of National Statistics [ONS], 2002).

## Risk factors associated with the development of COPD

The most significant risk factor for developing COPD is exposure to tobacco smoke, in that 80–90% of all cases are attributable to smoking (American Thoracic Society, 1995). More recently, it has been shown that 90% of people with COPD have a history of more than 20 pack years (Bellamy and Booker, 2003). (It should be noted, however, that only 15% of smokers develop COPD.) A pack year is a term used to describe the number of cigarettes a person has smoked over a lifetime. One pack year is defined as 20 manufactured cigarettes (one pack) smoked for one year. For example, a person who smokes 30 cigarettes per day for 26 years will have a history of 39 pack years (Bellamy and Booker, 2003):

• 1 pack per day x 26 years = 26 pack years
• ½ pack per day x 26 years = 13 pack years
• 26 pack years + 13 pack years = 39 pack years.

While much of the literature refers to cigarette smoking, the use of tobacco equally includes the one million pipe and cigar smokers in the UK (ASH, 2006). Furthermore, research indicates that passive smoking is a huge risk factor and could be responsible for in excess of 1.9 million deaths from COPD among non-smokers in China, and that susceptibility to the disease could be established *in utero* (Yin et al, 2007). Indeed, the global burden of COPD is increasing and projected to be the third leading cause of death and the fifth leading cause of disability worldwide by 2020 (Mannino et al, 2002).

The UK mortality rate attributable to COPD for 2002 (Office for National Statistics [ONS], 2002) indicates a lower death rate for women by some 10%. In the USA, however, the number of women dying from COPD surpasses that of men. It has been suggested that increased tobacco use in women explains some of this increase of COPD prevalence (Han et al, 2007). In the UK, the use of hand-rolled cigarettes has increased by 14%

among women, compared with just 2% 15 years ago. The key issue arising from the American data is that women may be at greater risk of smoking-induced lung function impairment, dyspnoea and poorer health status for the same level of tobacco exposure as men. Furthermore, suggest Han et al (2007), not only are the manifestations of the disease different in men and women, but the risk factors, symptoms, disease progression and even diagnosis, are markedly different between the sexes. Han et al (2007) note that one of the most significant differences in the manifestation of COPD is that women tend to develop more airway obstruction, whereas men tend to develop a more emphysematic manifestation.

There may be many reasons for these differences; behaviour, exposure to biomass fuels used for cooking in many parts of the world, and women taking their place in the industrial and manufacturing environments. COPD can develop over decades and a substantial number of current cases may be traced back to the rising smoking epidemic among women in the 1950s. There is also evidence indicating that female smokers seem to have more difficulty quitting (McEwan et al, 2006); all or none of these factors may prove to be valid. What is apparently clear from the research so far is that women seem to be more susceptible to developing COPD from exposure to cigarette smoke, but they also predominate among those COPD patients who have never smoked, and may have gender-linked factors that predispose them to developing the disease (Han et al, 2007). An example of this is alpha 1-antitrypsin deficiency. Alpha 1-antitrypsin is a protein that is produced mainly in the liver and its primary function is to protect the lungs from neutrophil elastase, which, if left unchecked, can destroy healthy lung tissue.

Other risks which may predispose to developing COPD include: exposure to indoor air pollution from cooking and heating; occupational hazards such as coal and wood dust irritants, fumes, and vapours; tuberculosis; age; poor airway function at birth; and cured meats (nitrites used to preserve the meats may cause structural changes to the lung resembling emphysema) (Jiang et al, 2007). Although smoking remains the single most significant cause of COPD, research suggests that there are many other factors that may result in an increased risk of developing the disease (Barnes, 2007).

---

### Reflection

- Consider the impact smoking has on the development of COPD
- How might you educate a patient about the risk of smoking?
- How might you support patients to give up smoking?

# How might the patient present?

Patients with COPD are usually found to be over 35 years of age, and often present with at least one risk factor (generally smoking), together with one or more of the following (NICE, 2004):

- A chronic cough (may not always be productive and may be described as a smokers cough)
- Regular sputum production
- Exertional dyspnoea (that is, breathlessness with exercise)
- Wheeze.

Patients may or may not have a smoking history and may complain of their symptoms worsening over the years. Some may report a seasonal worsening of their symptoms, usually during the winter months, or perhaps after a cold. The more severe the case, the greater the likelihood of the patient complaining of breathlessness on a daily basis and the normal activities of daily living becoming more difficult to sustain.

The Medical Research Council (MRC) has produced a dyspnoea scale, which lists five grades of severity (Fletcher et al, 1959):

*Grade*    *Degree of breathlessness related to activities*
1.      Not troubled by breathlessness except on strenuous exercise
2.      Short of breath when hurrying or walking up a slight hill
3.      Walks slower than contemporaries on level ground because of breathlessness, or has to stop for breath when walking at own pace
4.      Stops for breath after walking about 100 m or after a few minutes on level ground
5.      Too breathless to leave the house, or breathless when dressing or undressing.

There are other dyspnoea classification scales which may be of benefit, such as the New York Heart Association Dyspnoea Scale, which lists four grades of disability and includes the consideration of other daily living activities as a measure. However, it is the MRC scale that NICE (2004) recommend as a common standard of dyspnoea measure.

---

**Reflection**

- Consider the impact of breathlessness on lifestyle and quality of life
- How might this differ for younger patients, and elderly patients?

---

## How might patients feel?

Patients may describe to you a picture of reduced activity, lifestyle change or adaption in order to minimize the experience of dyspnoea. The unfortunate result of these and other misplaced coping strategies is a decline in physical fitness, reduced stamina, and dyspnoea triggered with ever-decreasing levels of activity. Note must always be taken of other symptoms which may be present in considering a diagnosis of COPD:

- Weight-loss and anorexia are often seen as the condition progresses. The patient may experience difficulty in eating and breathing at the same time. However, weight-loss may present as an early symptom in the event of low mood or depressive illness
- Effort intolerance and fatigue as a result of decreased levels of oxygen in the blood (hypoxia) caused by a narrowing of the airways, which will compromise the distribution of air within the lungs. This results in poor gaseous exchange and a low peripheral arterial oxygen content ($PaO_2$)
- Tiredness and general debility as a result of the increased physical demands required to breathe; inspiratory and expiratory muscle weakness play an important role in the symptoms associated with COPD, not least the need to increasingly depend on the use of accessory muscles to inflate the lungs
- Muscle weakness. Wasting of extremity fat-free mass is commonly found in COPD patients (Engelen et al, 2000) and is usually attributed to a general physical de-conditioning process and poor nutrition. It may also be attributed to circulating cytokines, proteins involved with the communication between lymphocytes and macrophages, and responsible for regulating a variety of immune and inflammatory responses. Owing to the complexity of the processes involved, the host defence and immunity response may become exaggerated and misdirected
- General aches and pains, which may be associated with other comorbidities, for example chest pain in cardiac-related complications or musculoskeletal strain

- Anxiety, panic attacks and depression. The brain uses 40% of the oxygen we breathe, but a reduced supply of oxygen causing hypoxia is associated with cognitive impairment and depression. Compromised breathing may be one of the reasons that the incidence of depression is higher in COPD than in other chronic conditions (Sharma, 2005). Other contributing factors may include social isolation, loneliness, managing the feelings of those near and dear, and the contemplation of end-of-life issues
- Oedema, if present, may present as ankle swelling and may be described by the patient as having swollen or puffy ankles (peripheral oedema). Peripheral oedema in the COPD patient is usually associated with congestive or right-sided heart failure (*cor pulmonale*). Fluid typically rests in the legs and ankles during the day in the ambulant patient, or if the patient is upright. At night, when the patient is recumbent, the fluid is reabsorbed, increasing the total blood volume and blood pressure and leading to pulmonary hypertension and the accumulation of fluid in the lungs (pulmonary oedema)
- Poor and disturbed sleep. The patient may describe waking suddenly from sleep with a sensation of acute breathlessness, wheezing and/or choking. He/she may report that this is relieved by sitting up (but not as quickly as in simple orthopnoea) or standing at an open window. Such information may lead you to consider issues of paroxysmal nocturnal dyspnoea (PND)
- Cough. This may or may not be chronic or productive and may simply be dismissed as an early morning or a winter smokers' cough by the patient
- Sputum. While sputum production and an accompanying cough can be a symptom of many conditions, COPD is frequently characterized by the production of variable amounts of sputum, which may differ in colour and consistency, from white and frothy to mucopurulent (containing both mucus and pus).

### What more could you find out about the patient's condition and how might you do it?

In providing effective and considered care to the patient, the nurse must develop good communication skills. These are paramount to developing a rapport with the patient and his/her carers, as are compassion, confidence and professionalism, to be able to usefully evaluate the patient's condition and concerns in detail. Effective listening skills, the appropriate use of non-verbal communication (Lugton, 2002), keen observation, recognizing both the normal and the abnormal, and being able to take a meaningful nursing and social history, will help to make the patient feel more comfortable and confident in discussing his/her condition. The more information the patient provides, the quicker and more likely you will be able to deliver effective treatment.

The patient's history will comprise the actual complaint(s) and any other information you have been able to collect through observation, examination, focused questioning, and initial clinical and physical tests and measurements. Once this information has been gathered, it will be possible to evaluate the impact of his/her symptoms on his/her life, and those of his/her family and/or carers.

Just as importantly, during the course of training and education the nurse will learn how to undertake a relevant physical examination. This can be supplemented by close observation, self-directed study and appropriate questioning of examining nurse specialists and doctors.

## What might you usefully ask and observe of the patient?

### Cough

You may observe characteristic COPD symptoms such as a productive cough; ask the patient about the nature of the cough:

- Is the cough acute or chronic? Is it of less than two months duration or more?
- If less than two months, think about upper respiratory infections and allergies
- If more than two months, think about more intrinsic lung disease, but also gastrointestinal and cardiac problems
- Is the patient taking any medication, for example angiotensin converting enzyme (ACE) inhibitors, that may cause the cough?
- If the cough is chronic, ask about timing. Is it triggered by certain times of the day, month or year? Ask about exacerbating factors such as smoking or exposure to polluted environments
- Is the cough productive? Not all patients are able to expectorate sputum, but this does not mean that it isn't there and there isn't an infection.

### Sputum

Ask the patient whether there has been any change or variation in sputum:

- Volume. Any change from the norm may be the first indication
  of an exacerbation caused by bacterial or viral infections, continued
  smoking or other environmental pollution, including passive
  smoking, smog, occupational hazards, wood and coal dust,
  for example
- Colour. White and frothy usually indicates that the patient is
  infection-free. However, if it is copious in volume and saliva-like
  it may indicate a bronchoalveolar carcinoma. Foamy and pink-tinged
  may indicate pulmonary oedema and heart failure, while frank
  blood (haemoptysis) may indicate bronchitis or bronchiectasis, or
  some other serious condition that may require urgent investigation
  and treatment
- Consistency. Sputum can be divided into three basic types: serous is
  runny and clear (serous sputum is rarely bacterial); mucoid is sticky
  (viscous) and clear; or mucopurulent/purulent is usually yellow or
  green in colour, but may also be grey. If the patient is dehydrated, the
  sputum is likely to be viscous and may be difficult to expectorate
- Taste and smell. The patient may be reluctant to raise this matter, but
  it is important to ask the question as it may indicate the presence of
  an anaerobic infection.

### Diet and nutrition

Ask the patient or carer(s) (with the patient's permission) whether there
has been any change in diet or appetite. COPD patients may be
malnourished, especially if he/she finds that eating makes him/her feel
breathless. Ask the patient whether there are any foods that he/she finds
particularly enjoyable or easy to eat. Encourage small, regular meals
and snacks, and the avoidance of gas-forming foods and drinks, as these
may cause abdominal distension and compromise lung space and therefore
lung function.

### Bowel and bladder management

Ask the patient to describe his/her normal bowel habits including frequency,
consistency, flatulence, and whether anything has changed recently. Items
of interest may include change in diet, medication that could cause a
constipatory or loose bowel syndrome effect, both of which may cause
abdominal distension and compromise the patient's breathing. A loaded
bowel can also cause difficulty in micturition, resulting in the patient
having to reduce fluid intake in order to manage bladder discomfort, with
predictable consequences arising from dehydration.

## Medication

Enquire what medication the patient is taking, both prescribed and over-the-counter. Ask the patient to show you any medication that he/she has, how it is taken and how often. Check this information against the prescribing instructions on the packaging. Ask whether there are any medications that he/she is prescribed but not currently taking. If using inhalers, ask about the frequency of use and check inhaler technique. Lack of concordance is probably the most important patient-related drug therapy problem, leading to unnecessary suffering and therapy failure (Marinker, 1997).

## Mental health

Actively listen to and note any patient concerns and problems as this may help to explain and understand the nature of some of the patient's current symptoms, such as breathlessness, anxiety, loss of appetite, tearfulness, mood or uncharacteristic behaviour.

Other issues to be aware of are that hypoxia may present as a confusional or depressed state, and that emotions can have a profound effect on breathing patterns which, if not effectively managed, may trigger a spiral of panic and anxiety.

## Breathing

Note the patient's breathing pattern. Ask whether it has changed significantly and whether he/she can link the change to an event. Once you have established a rapport with the patient and reassured him/her, try to count the respiratory rate and the nature of breathing. Is it slow and deep, or rapid and short? Is there pain experienced on breathing? Ask how many pillows the patient sleeps on at night, and does he/she experience any difficulties if he/she slips down the bed during sleep? Does the patient use home oxygen and if so, for how long per day, and at what litre rate and percentage? Who set the rate and has it been altered recently and by whom?

On occasion, you will find that a well-meaning patient or carer has significantly and without medical advice increased the oxygen delivery rate causing symptoms of respiratory depression. Assess how much exercise the patient takes daily, and whether this has reduced and for what reason.

The key point in asking the patient these and other searching questions is to ascertain what changes he/she is experiencing or has made from what he/she might consider to be the norm. Do not forget that changes in breathing pattern in the COPD patient may be due to other new or associated comorbidities.

## The physical examination

While the principle and subsequent physical examination of the patient will be carried out by medical staff, medical students and specialist/senior nurses, there is no reason why a junior or student nurse with the informed consent of the patient should not collect and record clinical data arising from a basic physical examination of the patient. Any findings should be discussed with the doctor or a senior nurse. This exercise might include:

- Generally observe the patient and listen for any untoward sounds, cough, breathing, wheeze and respiratory rate and breathlessness (it can be difficult to ascertain whether the symptom is a consequence of physical, psychological, social or spiritual circumstances) (McLeod, 2005). You may want to use the MRC dyspnoea scale to assist you in your assessment
- Note any smells or odours, including tobacco smoke, vomit and malodorous breath
- Note the patient's colour generally and at the extremities
- Examine the hands, noting any clubbing of the fingers, cyanosis, tremor, muscle wasting and tobacco staining
- Note the pulse rate and rhythm. These may be altered in respiratory disease. Chest infections may cause a tachycardia (typically a ventricular heart rate of greater than 100 beats per minute), whereas a large bounding pulse might be a sign of carbon dioxide retention suggesting respiratory failure
- Does the patient's chest expand equally on inhaling and does it deflate equally on exhaling? Is the patient using accessory muscles when breathing and does the he/she look distressed?
- Does the patient appear well nourished or not? Ask about diet
- Examine the feet and legs, noting muscle wasting, cyanosis (blue colouration of the blood/tissue, indicating an oxygen saturation of 85–90%), and oedema
- Record the patient's oxygen saturation using a pulse oximeter. Ensure that the patient's hands are warm as cold fingers or poor circulation may lead to an underestimated $O_2$ saturation level. Nail varnish and skin stained by tobacco smoke or other stains will impair the ability of the pulse oximeter to read the pigment colour of the blood. Ask the patient whether he/she has recently smoked or been exposed to tobacco smoke—pulse oximeters cannot differentiate

between carbon dioxide and oxygen. If the patient has recently smoked it can take 24 hours for high $CO_2$ levels to be removed from the blood
- Mobility/exercise. Ask the patient whether he/she takes regular exercise and describe what he/she does, how often, whether he/she gets out of breath by the end of his exercise. Ask how far the patient can walk until he/she becomes a little breathless.

## Diagnosis

A diagnosis of COPD will be made on clinical features and symptoms, many of which have been described in this chapter, together with evidence obtained from spirometry tests, which measure how quickly the patient can force air out of the lungs and therefore the severity of obstruction in the airways. Different lung conditions produce different results and this test helps to separate COPD from other lung diseases.

## Treatment

There are a range of therapies and interventions that may help to relieve the patient's symptoms, including:

- Bronchodilators. These drugs are often administered via inhaler or nebulizer, but not exclusively. The aim is to relieve wheezing and breathlessness by relaxing the bronchioles so that the air flows into them more easily
- Steroids. A small maintenance dose of oral corticosteroids may help if the patient is wheezy or breathless at times when bronchodilators are not sufficiently effective. The dose is often increased for a limited time to treat exacerbations
- Mucolytics. These break down viscid secretions in the lung, making it easier for the patient to expectorate sputum
- Oxygen therapy. In the event of the condition becoming severe, the patient may develop low oxygen levels, therefore this type of therapy may be prescribed to address symptoms of hypoxia. This may be short- or long-term via bottles or a concentrator
- Anxiolytics. These may help to reduce anxiety and panic attacks with associated hyperventilation and sensation of breathlessness. Some of these drugs are known to depress respiration and the potential advantages of using them should be weighed against the possible risks (Davis, 1997)

- Opiates, particularly in end-stage care where bronchodilators fail to relieve symptoms. Small doses of an opiate may relieve anxiety, but again the risk of respiratory depression will need to be considered
- Physical therapies. Using the expertise of physiotherapists and occupational therapists to address exercise programmes, chest clearance and breathing techniques. Challenges arising from the activities of daily living can be explored together with anxiety management and relaxation skills
- Surgery. For some patients surgery may be an option where the diseased area of the lung is removed to allow it to function more effectively.

## Exacerbation

COPD is, by its nature, a very unstable condition. Patients are prone to episodes of sustained worsening of their symptoms, which are beyond their normal day-to-day variations and are acute in onset. Symptoms include (NICE, 2004):

- Worsening breathlessness
- Cough
- Increase in sputum production, colour and nature
- Change in ability to carry out daily activities.

Exacerbations may be experienced at any stage of COPD and patients may experience two or more exacerbations per year (O'Reilly et al, 2004). As patients approach the palliative stage of their illness, the more frequently exacerbations are likely to occur. These patients, with each successive exacerbation, may not recover the pre-exacerbation lung function and deteriorate with increasing debility.

Exacerbations can be serious and life-threatening. Prompt and effective treatment is the key to the effective management of the condition. Many patients are now safely and cost-effectively managed in their own homes by experienced health professionals (Burton, 2004; British Pharmaceutical Conference [BPC], 2008), who will review the patient's pharmacological and/or therapy options by introducing, increasing and optimizing—as required—the use of the variety of medications and services available. In some cases, it is necessary to admit the patient to hospital to receive treatments that are not readily available in the community setting.

## Self-help

The effective management of COPD requires the active participation of the patient in an agreed care and life strategy. This must include:

- Removing factors that will worsen the condition, such as smoking and exposure to a smoky or polluted environment, including high pollen levels
- Balanced exercise and rest periods — developing a lifestyle that does not revolve around illness, but adjusts to it
- Participating in pulmonary rehabilitation programmes
- Weight-loss as required
- Sensible alcohol consumption
- Understanding COPD and how to manage symptoms
- Concordance with prescribed medication, including oxygen therapy
- Pneumococcal vaccination and an annual influenza vaccination should be sought (Poole et al, 2006)
- Avoiding exposure to viral and bacterial infections
- A written self-management plan agreed with a responsible health professional to enable the prompt treatment of an exacerbation. This will often include antibiotics and corticosteroids prescribed in anticipation of such an eventuality
- As appropriate, an agreed end-of-life plan.

## Case study

Agnes is a 76-year-old retired office worker with a diagnosis of COPD. She lives independently with her pet dog in an older persons' local authority bungalow. She smokes 10–15 cigarettes per day and had a 90 pack year history up to 18 months ago. She was thought to be concordant with her prescribed medication, which was delivered from repeat prescriptions by the local pharmacy. Agnes uses an oxygen concentrator to deliver 2L/min of oxygen 24 hours every day. It has been one year since Agnes walked outside with her wheeled walking aid and portable oxygen. Her GP undertook a home visit at the request of the patient, who was complaining of excessive and viscid sputum, which she was having difficulty in expectorating. At this time, he advised Agnes that if she didn't stop smoking he would have the oxygen concentrator removed from her home because of the fire risk. The community matron was asked by the GP to assess the patient's continued risks to herself and her neighbours.

## Problem

With the patient's agreement, the community matron carried out an assessment of the patient's circumstances and found that:

- Agnes was reluctant to call her GP for fear that her concentrator would be removed
- She had reduced her smoking habit unaided over the past 18 months, but still felt the need to smoke when stressed and agitated
- She had a history of depressive illness and had stopped taking her antidepressants six months ago 'because they were not doing anything'. (She has not told her GP and still receives monthly repeat prescriptions)
- She felt she had little control of her life and was not going to entertain anyone coming in to her home and 'telling her what to do'
- Agnes had a poor sleep pattern owing to difficulty in expectorating sputum, an uncontrolled cough, and an inability to maintain an upright position in bed throughout the night
- Her activity and mobility had decreased owing to breathlessness and resultant anxiety. She had also fallen in her home on two occasions in the past six months.

## Diagnosis

- Chronic obstruction of the airways exacerbated by smoking
- Ineffective airway clearance related to viscid sputum causing uncontrolled cough, poor sleep pattern, dyspnoea and anxiety
- Risk of a bacterial chest infection resulting from mucoid congestion
- Unresolved long-standing depressive illness
- Fatigue owing to inadequate oxygenation for activities compromised by smoking, poor nutrition and fluid intake
- Risk of cognitive impairment and low mood compromised by hypoxia
- Other risks include fire, falls and social isolation.

---

### Reflection

- Look at the case history
- What do you think are Agnes' main priorities?
- What are the nurses' main priorities?
- What are possible effective management strategies in this case?

---

## *Nursing intervention*

Following a basic physical examination, evaluation of medications and recent medical and social history, the following strategy was adopted. With the agreement of the patient, discussions and negotiations took place during a three-week period to explore possible management strategies for maintaining and improving Agnes's independence and confidence. Agnes appreciated that it was dangerous to smoke while using oxygen and agreed with immediate effect to:

- Turn off all oxygen, remove her nasal cannulae and move to the kitchen or patio (weather permitting) before smoking
- Not smoke where there were bottled or other oxygen supplies
- Keep her cigarettes, matches and ash tray in the kitchen.

The community matron undertook to assure the GP of these undertakings. Agnes was reassured as to the genuine care and concern of her GP and agreed that the community matron would collaborate with him in her continuing care, and:

- Further curb her smoking by using a nicotine inhalator and nicotine replacement patches. Besides addressing her cravings, the inhalator device would give her something to do with her hands and therefore reduce displacement activity. Agnes understands that the consequence of her continued smoking is an accelerated and progressive decline into respiratory failure
- Agnes agreed to continue with her other medication as prescribed and increase the use of saline inhalations via her nebulizer. Her inhaler device technique was assessed and corrected.
- An electric bed with 4-section profiling was ordered to give Agnes more control of her posture and a firmer base on which to sleep
- Agnes agreed that the community matron, in discussion with her GP, re-prescribe her previous antidepressant medication at a higher dose and monitor her progress
- A falls assessment was undertaken and recommendations made to minimize risks.

Agnes declined an offer to attend a pulmonary rehabilitation programme, but was happy to meet with a respiratory nurse specialist for instruction and support with breathing exercises and coughing techniques, with an ongoing shared-care approach. Agnes continues to receive the support of her community matron and respiratory nurse specialist, who share visits every two weeks on unspecified days in order to rule out selective smoking concordance on visit days. Agnes has further reduced her smoking, but still insists on 'enjoying a fag' in relative safety. Her mental health status has significantly improved over the past six months. She still hasn't ventured out beyond her garden, but is entertaining friends and family at home. She has been fall-free and her oxygen saturation levels are steady at 94% on oxygen. Agnes has an agreed care plan in place and emergency medication to address her out-of-hours needs as they arise.

The key to achieving a measure of success in this case was the willingness of the primary care health professionals to recognize the patient's needs and to accommodate them without compromising on safety, in order to achieve the optimum outcome in the home.

## Conclusion

The most effective strategy for the management of COPD is to limit cigarette smoking. However, so many people have been damaged by cigarettes that it will take decades to wipe out the effects on the health of the nation. That is, of course, supposing that cigarettes were to disappear tomorrow. There are still 10 million people in the UK who continue to smoke despite national information and education strategies, and as many as 450 children take up the habit every day (Calverley, 2005). As a result, upwards of 238 000 deaths will continue to be attributed to COPD each year posing a huge challenge to the NHS (ASH, 2006).

---

### Activities

- Spend some time with a respiratory nurse specialist both on the ward and in the clinic. Ask whether you can (with the permission of the patient) undertake a supervised examination of the patient as described in this chapter
- Having done so, discuss the exercise with your mentor and the patient. Record your clinical and nursing reflections
- Spend some time with a community matron while on your community placement. Discuss how the nurse's role in striving to provide planned and symptomatic relief for patients in the community has and will continue to change
- Discuss with your mentors the palliative and end-of-life planning needs of patients with non-malignant terminal illness and identify any local shortfalls

---

Action on Smoking and Health (2006) Smoking statistics: illness and death. http://tinyurl. com/yk4a4ut (accessed 9 December 2009)

Araya J, Cambier S, Markovics JA et al (2007) Squamous metoplasia amplifies pathologic epithelial-mesenchymal interactions in COPD patients. *J Clin Invest* **117**(11): 3551–62

Barnes PJ (2000) Chronic obstructive pulmonary disease. *N Engl J Med* **343**(4): 269–80

Barnes PJ (2007) Chronic obstructive pulmonary disease: a growing but neglected global epidemic. *PLoS Med* **4**(5): e112

Bellamy D, Booker R (2003) *Chronic Obstructive Pulmonary Disease in Primary Care: All You Need to Know to Manage COPD in Your Practice.* 3rd edn. Class Health, London

Bobadilla A, Guerra S, Sherrill D, Barbee R (2002) How accurate is the self-reported diagnosis of chronic bronchitis? *Chest* **122**(4): 1234–9

Bourke SJ (2003) *Respiratory Medicine.* 6th edn. Blackwell, Oxford

British Pharmaceutical Conference (2008) Pharmacists reduce hospital visits for respiratory patients. 7–9 September, Manchester Central

Burton S (2004) Early discharge of people with chronic obstructive pulmonary disease. *Nurs Times* **100**(6): 65–7

Calverley PC (2005) COPD. In: British Lung Foundation, *Lung Report III — Casting a shadow over the nation's health.* http://tinyurl.com/n9r3db (accessed 14 October 2009)

Davis CL (1997) ABC of palliative care. Breathlessness, cough and other respiratory problems. *BMJ* **315**(7113): 931–4

Dewar M, Curry RW Jr (2006) Chronic obstructive pulmonary disease: diagnostic considerations. *Am Fam Physician* **73**(4): 669–76

Engelen MP, Schols AM, Does JD, Wouters EF (2000) Skeletal muscle weakness is associated with wasting of extremity fat-free mass but not with airflow obstruction in patients with chronic obstructive pulmonary disease. *Am J Clin Nutr* **71**(3): 733–8

Fletcher CM, Elmes PC, Fairbairn AS, Wood CH (1959) The significance of respiratory symptoms and the diagnosis of chronic bronchitis in a working population. *BMJ* **2**(5147): 257–66

GOLD (2004) Global Strategy for the Diagnosis, Management, and Prevention of COPD. Executive summary. http://tinyurl.com/ygxa99r (accessed 14 October 2009)

Han MK, Postma D, Mannino DM et al (2007) Gender and chronic obstructive airways disease. *Am J Respir Crit Care Med* **176**: 1179–84

Holleman DR Jr, Simel DL (1995) Does the clinical examination predict airflow limitation ? *JAMA* **273**(4): 313–9

Jiang R, Paik DC, Hankinson JL, Barr RG (2007) Cured meat consumption, lung function, and chronic obstructive pulmonary disease among United States adults. *Am J Respir Crit Care Med* **175**(8): 798–804

Lugton J (2002) *Communicating with Dying People and Their Relatives.* Radcliffe

Publishing, London

Mannino DM, Homa DM, Akinbami LJ, Ford ES, Redd SC (2002) Chronic obstructive airways disease surveillance—United States, 1971–2000. *Respir Care* **47**(10): 1184–99

Marinker M (1997) *From Compliance to Concordance: Achieving shared goals in medicine taking*. Royal Pharmacological Society, London

McLeod R (2005) Dyspnoea management: psychosocial therapies. In: Ahmedzai S, Muers MF. eds, *Supportive Care in Respiratory Disease*. Oxford University Press, USA

McEwan A, Hajek P, McRobbie P, West R (2006) *Manual of Smoking Cessation: A Guide for Counsellors and Practitioners*. Blackwell Publishing, Oxford

Minkoff NB (2005) Analysis of the current care model of the COPD patient: a health outcomes assessment and economic evaluation. *J Manag Care Pharm* **2**(6 Suppl A): S3–7

NCCCC (2004) Chronic obstructive pulmonary disease: national guidelines for the management of chronic obstructive pulmonary disease in adults in primary and secondary care. *Thorax* **59**(Suppl 1): 1–232

New York Heart Association (NYHA) Functional Classification Scale. www.hom.org/clinical/nyha.asp (accessed 9 December 2009)

The NHS Information Centre (2008) Statistics on NHS Stop Smoking Services: England, April 2007 to March 2008. http://tinyurl.com/5l2ev5 (accessed 14 October 2009)

NICE (2004) Management of chronic obstructive pulmonary disease in adults in primary and secondary care. http://guidance.nice.org.uk/CG12 (accessed 9 December 2009)

Office for National Statistics (2002) Mortality Statistics 2002. General Register Office for Scotland, 2002; Registrar General Northern Ireland. Annual Report Statistics and Research Agency, 2002. http://tinyurl.com/yl4zo9r (accessed 26 November 2009)

O'Reilly JF, Williams AE, Rice L, Holt K (2004) Incidence and impact of healthcare—defined exacerbations amongst a cohort of primary care COPD patients. European Respiratory Society Annual Congress, 4–8 September, Glasgow

Petty TL (2002) COPD in perspective. *Chest* **121**(5 Suppl): 116S–120S

Poole PJ, Chacko E, Wood-Baker RW, Cates CJ (2006) Influenza vaccine for patients with chronic obstructive pulmonary disease. *Cochrane Database Syst Rev* (1):CD002733

Puchelle E, Zahm JM, Tournier JM, Coraux C (2006) Airway epithelial repair regeneration and remodelling after injury in chronic obstructive pulmonary disease. *Proc Am Thorac Soc* **3**(8): 726–33

Rennard SI (2002) Overview of causes of COPD. New understanding of pathogenesis and mechanisms can guide future therapy. *Postgrad Med* **111**(6): 28–30, 33–4, 37–8

Sharma VP (2005) Overcoming Depression In COPD Part 1. http://mindpub.com/art550.htm (accessed 14 October 2009)

Tobacco Advisory Group (2000) *Nicotine Addiction in Britain. A Report of the Tobacco*

*Advisory Group of the Royal College of Physicians*. RCP, London

Viegi G, Scognamiglio A, Baldacci S, Pistelli F, Carrozzi L (2001) Epidemiology of chronic obstructive pulmonary disease (COPD). *Respiration* **68**(1): 4–19

Yin P, Jiang CQ, Cheng KK et al (2007) Passive smoking exposure and risk of COPD among adults in China: the Guangzhou Biobank Cohort Study. *Lancet* **370**(9589): 751–7

## Suggested reading and useful websites

Action on Smoking and Health (ASH) www.ash.org.uk (accessed 14 October 2009)

Barnett M (2006) Providing palliative care in end-stage COPD within primary care. *Br J Community Nurs* **20**(3): 30–4

Bowers S (2004) COPD is not a death sentence. *Lancet* **364**(9437): 896

British Thoracic Society (2006) The Burden of Lung Disease. 2nd edn. http://tinyurl.com/yzorjmp (accessed 14 October 2009)

Cox N (2007) Respiratory System. In: Cox NLT, Roper TA. eds, *Clinical Skills*. Oxford University Press, Oxford

Reilly S (2007) LTOT in COPD and the care of patients in the home. *Nursing in Practice* **38**: 63–6

# CHAPTER 6

# Rheumatoid arthritis

*Karen Ford*

Arthritis is one of the most common long-term conditions. Approximately 8.8 million people in the UK have a diagnosis of arthritis, 400 000 of which will have rheumatoid arthritis (RA) (Arthritis Research Campaign [ARC], 2009). The National Audit Office (NAO) (2009) suggests that this figure is much higher, with 700 000 cases in the UK. This chapter explores the management of RA. By reading this chapter and reflecting on your own experiences, you should achieve the following learning outcomes:

* Raising your awareness of the importance of early diagnosis
* Appreciating the importance of the nurse's role in support
  and care provision
* Understanding the psychosocial impact of RA
* Increasing your knowledge of the variety of management
  options available
* Identifying where health promotion and health education strategies
  can be used.

RA is not a modern condition—there is evidence that it has affected humans since before the 14th century (Blondiaux et al, 1997). It is different to osteoarthritis, which is a degenerative disorder of wear and tear to the joints, affecting the larger joints in the body that have been involved in weight-bearing (Lucas, 2006).

RA is an autoimmune condition of the connective tissue, in which the body attacks its own tissue (National Institute for Health and Clinical Excellence [NICE], 2009). It is the second most common form of arthritis (osteoarthritis is the most common), affecting between one and three people per hundred and beginning at any age, with three quarters of sufferers being women (ARC, 2007). The joints affected vary between individuals, but the hands and feet are commonly affected on both sides of the body (ARC, 2007). In contrast to osteoarthritis, smaller joints in the body tend to be affected by RA (Lucas, 2006).

# Aetiology and physiology

The exact cause of RA is unknown, but there is a genetic component (Ryan and Oliver, 2002). This is thought to combine with an environmental trigger. The trigger could be an infection, stress (Burbage, 2008), or trauma (Lucas, 2006). This initiates inflammatory processes caused by the production of antibodies, which attack the body's joints, further leading to joint damage and affecting other organs and specific systems within the body. In the joint, smooth cartilage covers the ends of the bones, allowing it to move friction-free against the opposing bone. A membrane called the synovium surrounds the joint, which produces a small amount of synovial fluid to lubricate the cartilage and keep it slippery, facilitating smooth movement. In RA, the synovium around the joint becomes thicker, with increasing cell infiltration. This causes fluid to accumulate around the joint and the joint becomes swollen, hot and painful. The pain and swelling is a result of the release of prostaglandins and other chemical mediators that cause progressive damage to the joints (Greenstein et al, 2004). RA is characterized by symmetrical small joints of the hands and feet being affected, but larger joints can also be damaged (Ryan and Oliver, 2002). Although RA is considered to be a musculoskeletal condition, it can affect other important systems of the body, such as the eyes, blood, nervous system, and cardiovascular and respiratory systems (Burbage, 2008). RA is therefore a potentially debilitating, chronic condition.

# Signs and symptoms

To determine whether someone has RA, a history of symptoms is useful. Although it can occur at any age, it usually affects people at 30 or 40 years of age (Lucas, 2006). Approximately 400 000 adults in the UK have RA (Symmons et al, 2002), with a further 20 000 new cases diagnosed every year (ARC, 2006). Adults may experience: a sudden and acute onset of symptoms with many joints affected, stiffness in the joint in the morning, weight-loss, loss of appetite, symptoms of anaemia, and mild pyrexia (Lucas, 2006).

To identify the early signs and symptoms and confirm a diagnosis of RA, the revised classification guidance originally produced by the American Rheumatism Association is useful (Arnett et al, 1988). The individual must have at least four of the following signs, the first four of which must be present for over six weeks:

- Morning stiffness lasting for one hour before improvement
- Soft tissue swelling of three or more joints

- Swelling of the middle joints of the fingers, knuckles and wrist joints
- Symmetric arthritis
- Subcutaneous nodules
- Positive test for rheumatoid factor (complex of immunoglobulin G and anti-immunoglobulin G formed in joints in RA)
- X-ray changes of bone thinning in the hand or wrist joints.

An essential element of nursing care provision involves early diagnosis (Burbage, 2008). This is central to the subsequent management of the condition and is important to dispel the false assumption that nothing can be done to help people with RA (Oliver et al, 2008). It is a fact that patients who have RA can visit their GP up to four times before a diagnosis of RA is made (NAO, 2009), hence the important role the nurse can perform in the early diagnosis and appropriate referral.

Nurses working in primary care can also offer relief of symptoms and assess the psychosocial needs of the person, thereby facilitating the preservation of joint function and preventing long-term damage or deformity. Other goals should include the support of self-care to maximize independence and positively influence quality of life. Nurses in primary care can also help to maintain the remission experienced by RA sufferers. One of the only identifiable triggers for RA is smoking, which is linked to the emerging genetic susceptibility that is being revealed as a consequence of the Human Genome Project (Huizinga, 2003).

Health care needs to be accessible in line with the Department of Health's (DH) *Musculoskeletal Services Framework* (DH, 2006). The DH suggests three models: disease management, case management, and supporting wellbeing and self-care. The models promote the concept of a person with RA being able to access a range of services from the multidisciplinary team to empower them to help themselves, thereby retaining control over their own health. This approach promotes independence, particularly following episodes of care in hospital, and emphasizes the importance of nurses working in primary care and the role they play in supporting individuals with RA to manage their condition as close to home as possible.

---

### Reflection

- Have you nursed anyone with RA?
- At what age did they first develop symptoms?
- What level of disability did they have?

---

The effects of RA can be overwhelming, with half of sufferers becoming registered disabled within three years of receiving their diagnosis. If the arthritis is very serious, it can shorten an individual's life expectancy by 10 years (Burbage, 2008). The economic cost of musculoskeletal conditions to society is significant—four out of 10 people with RA lose their jobs within five years of diagnosis, and one in seven give up work within a year of being diagnosed (ARC, 2009).

## Reaching a diagnosis

Diagnosis can be obtained using a variety of blood tests. The rheumatoid factor (RF) is present in 70–90% of cases, but can be absent for up to six months in the early diagnostic period (Ryan and Oliver, 2002). Other blood tests look for signs of the inflammatory process in the body: full blood count (FBC); urea and electrolytes; liver function test (LFT); erythrocyte sedimentation rate (ESR); or C-reactive protein (CRP). A new blood test, anti-cyclic citrullinated peptide antibody (anti-CCP), measures specific antibodies and can assist in the diagnostic process, particularly where there has been a negative RF test (Burbage, 2008). Other antibody studies may also be carried out. Symptoms are, however, the main decisive factor and should alert the nurse or doctor to the potential diagnosis of RA. Radiological evidence may reveal the condition and is useful to monitor disease progression.

Early referral to a specialist service for rheumatology is essential to reduce potential joint damage and progression of the disease in many cases. This corresponds to key recommendations from the European League Against Rheumatism (EULAR) (Combe et al, 2007). The nurse working in primary care has an important role to play in recognizing the early signs of RA to facilitate a specialist referral and halt the progression of the condition. Pain is usually the earliest symptom, varying in intensity and joint sites on different days. The individual may complain of feeling stiff in the mornings—as a person ages he/she may put this down to growing older. This 'morning stiffness' can last from a few minutes up to a few hours. Feeling the affected joints for signs of swelling and heat can help in the assessment process. The individual may tell the nurse that he/she is aware of a reduction in mobility. This may be highlighted by a reduction in the normal use of his/her hands, and this can assist the nurse to identify RA. Sometimes muscle weakness can occur and this in turn could lead to muscle wasting (atrophy). Joints may have lumps (nodules) around them. This is indicative of the underlying pathophysiology within the affected joints. Tendons may even rupture.

# Management and the nurse's role

The management of RA initially focuses on pain relief and support for the patient to modify his/her activity in a way that reduces pain but maximizes independence and function. The multidisciplinary team involved come from both primary and secondary care, with the patient and his/her family as part of this partnership. A health promotion model to consider is the client-centred approach (Ewles and Simnett, 2003), in which the client (patient) is integral to the decision-making process. Care and advice can then be tailored to individual circumstances with the aim of empowering the patient to achieve the best outcomes for him/herself. This is also conducive to a concordant approach in which the client/patient is a partner in his/her own care, sharing power with the health professionals (Weiss and Britten, 2003). This philosophy is more likely to achieve compliance and subsequent satisfaction for all.

## Pain control

Pain is a debilitating feature of RA. There are a variety of approaches that could be considered to effectively manage this, including pharmaceutical therapies, complementary therapies and surgical intervention (*Table 6.1*).

Disease-modifying anti-rheumatic drugs (DMARDs) are frontline therapies, either used alone or in combination with non-steroidal anti-inflammatory drugs (NSAIDs) and anti-inflammatory steroids. DMARDs slow the rate of the degenerative changes in the joints, delaying or preventing deformity of the hands and feet, as well as controlling the pain, stiffness and swelling in the joints (Greenstein et al, 2004). The DMARDs of choice are methotrexate and sulfasalazine. Other DMARDs include chloroquine, gold salts, and penicillamine (ARC, 2008; Joint Formulary Committee, 2009). Their action is to inhibit the immune system's effect on the joints, but it can take up to six months for their efficacy to reach the full potential (Greenstein et al, 2004). Folic acid will be given if methotrexate is used. These drugs can have severe adverse effects, so careful monitoring is required. In combination, individuals may also receive anti-inflammatory steroids in small dosages, often reserved for flare-ups or chronic RA as they can have adverse effects if used for long periods of time.

Sometimes flare-up management may be necessary to reduce the inflammation using NSAIDs, particularly the selective inhibitor of cylcooxygenase-2 (Cox-2) drugs. As NSAIDs do not address the problem of joint damage and have no effect on the cytokines, they are no longer used for frontline therapy (Greenstein et al, 2004). Recent research has been presented at the EULAR (Nursing Times, 2009), finding promising results to halt the

**Table 6.1 Possible management options**

| Drug category | Mode of action | Potential side-effects/ key considerations |
|---|---|---|
| Anti-inflammatory steroids, e.g. prednisolone, methylprednisolone | Suppression of inflammation | Diabetes, osteoporosis, Cushing's syndrome, gastrointestinal effects, water retention |
| NSAIDs, e.g. ibuprofen | Reduces production of prostaglandins by inhibition of enzyme cyclooxygenase-2 | Gastrointestinal discomfort, nausea and occasionally bleeding |
| DMARDs, e.g. | Inhibit the effects of the body's immune system | Can take up to 6 months to produce effect |
| chloroquine | Reduces morning stiffness, mode of action not clear | Retinal damage with prolonged treatment |
| penicillamine | Interferes with enzymes that attack the joints | Skin rashes, proteinuria, cytopenia |
| methotrexate | Antagonist of folic acid and is cytotoxic | Gastrointestinal upset, liver cirrhosis, pulmonary fibrosis |
| sulfasalazine | A combination of sulphonamide and salicylate suppress the rheumatoid process | Takes 3 months to produce effect. Less toxic than penicillamine, but regular blood tests and liver function tests needed |
| Biological DMARDs e.g. etanercept, abatacept, inlfiximab | Neutralize a cytokine involved in the inflammatory process | Not oral therapies. Fever and cold symptoms and skin rashes |
| rituximab | A monoclonal antibody causes lysis of B lymphocytes | Costly drugs. Used in combination with methotrexate where condition has not |

| | | responded to other DMARDs |
|---|---|---|
| Other DMARDs, e.g. azathiaprine, cylclophosphamide, cylosporin | Target specialized T-cells involved in rheumatoid inflammatory process | Gastrointestinal disturbance, renal and liver impairment, hypertension, immune suppression issues |

From: Greenstein et al (2004), Joint Formulary Committee (2009)
DMARDs=disease-modifying anti-rheumatic drugs;
NSAIDs=non-steroidal anti-inflammatory drugs

progression of RA by early administration of methotrexate and rituximab, a monoclonal antibody which causes lysis of B lymphocytes (Joint Formulary Committee, 2009). Non-opiod analgesics such as paracetamol may also have some benefit for pain management. It may be difficult for the person with RA to differentiate between pain and stiffness, however.

Adjuncts to drug therapy, such as hot or cold therapy or transcutaneous electrical nerve stimulation (TENS), can be tried or massage may benefit, although the evidence for this is anecdotal (Hill and Hale, 2004). Joint splinting may help reduce pain and deformity, or be useful at night for example, when the pain seems to worsen (Hill and Hale, 2004). Surgical interventions, including synovectomy, arthroplasty, osteotomy and arthrodesis, may also be necessary (Lucas, 2006). There are some herbal remedies available that have undergone randomized controlled trials, but these do not offer a complete solution and are poorly rated as a treatment option (ARC, 2008).

For the nurse, it is important to consider patient choice and the information he/she may require about the evidence supporting herbal remedies. There is always the potential for drug interactions with prescribed medication and herbal remedies. Others may seek complementary therapies such as acupuncture or a variety of other options, which they may find helpful to them individually. The nurse must remember not to recommend complementary therapies that he/she has not obtained a specialist qualification in. This is in line with nurse's professional accountability (Nursing and Midwifery Council [NMC], 2008), but can cause tension when endeavouring to support individual choice.

The emotional impact of pain is an important factor to consider when working with the person who has RA. Individuals respond differently to pain and the degree to which the patient wants to be free of the pain has an impact on the severity. Anger and the emotional impact of diagnosis will also play a part in the perception of pain (Niven, 2006). The nurse's role is one of providing information and assessing pain, including the use of a pain assessment tool. There are a number of tools available; a multidimensional tool which explores both the quantitative and qualitative aspect of pain may be more appropriate for example the brief pain inventory (Mann and Carr, 2009). This can help both nurse and client to monitor the efficacy of treatments, and therefore be positive for both parties in recognizing relief and severity. It is also paramount for the nurse to acknowledge the varying cultural perception of pain. The nurse's cultural view may minimize pain and the psychological distress it causes, or conversely the patient's cultural perspective may require regular verbalization of pain at odds with the nurse's approach (Gross and Kinnison, 2007). For the older person, it is important to remember the long-term impact that RA can have. A person who has lived with RA for many years will have learnt to cope and adapt to chronic pain and fatigue, making adjustments to their independence and mobility (Melanson and Downe-Wamboldt, 2003).

---

### Reflection

Think about a person who has RA. What impact does pain and reduced mobility have on the quality of life for:
- An older person?
- An individual of working age?

---

## Maintaining independence and optimizing wellbeing

The use of a nursing model, such as Orem's Self Care Model (2001), will enable the nurse to have a sound framework to support all aspects of care for the patient with RA. A self-care model may be the most appropriate to ensure the focus of promoting and maintaining independence is central to all care and support. For the elderly, it may be appropriate to consider a model of care that incorporates the self-determination required by the individual to cope with the chronic pain and gradual loss of function and independence (Löfman et al, 2008). It is important to consider the age of the individual, employment status, and whether he/she has a young family, in which case he/she may wish to continue their life as normally as possible. For the nurse, it may be more challenging to support a patient with an external locus of control, where he/she feels his/her health is governed from outside, having no say in their health and future progress of this chronic condition. To have an external locus of control implies that one does not have control over one's health and will, therefore, not take responsibility for making changes that would improve wellbeing (Niven, 2006). This implies that people with an internal locus will take charge of their health destiny.

Psychological and sociological theory can help the nurse to understand why a person acts the way that they do when they are unwell. If the nurse can encourage the individual to see the benefits of complying with medication in terms of reducing flare-ups and being independent for example, this has a positive benefit to both the patient and his/her family, through 'reasoned action and planned behaviour' (Niven, 2007). From an ethical perspective, the nurse must also respect the individual's autonomy (Edwards, 1996) and choice in how he/she manages his/her illness, which may conflict with the nurse's own views. The initial impact of the diagnosis can be devastating and providing evidence-based information will be vital at this time. The person with RA may have older family members with the condition and envisage the same pain and debility for themselves.

The stages of denial, anger, grief and acceptance (Hill and Hale, 2004) are often visited and revisited, and the nurse will need to be aware of this oscillation of feelings and offer support and understanding at these times. Again, information is key to explain the new treatment options available and the importance of early specialist intervention to minimize damage to the joints.

## Exercise and rest

Balancing activity and rest is important, together with advising the individual to use the larger joints rather than smaller ones in an endeavour to minimize damage. Muscle power may be reduced and changes may be required in the home or workplace to reduce stress on the joints and maximize activity and independence. For example, a seat that ejects, a raised toilet seat, or a workstation assessment to reduce effort. A bed that has a variable height may also be of benefit (Lucas, 2006). Hill and Hale (2004) outline the problems with washing and dressing, getting out of bed, preparing and eating food, caring for others, driving, and working. The key is to gradually encourage increasing activity and low-impact activities such as swimming, walking or dancing. The physiotherapist can teach specific ranges of movement exercises, which can be undertaken before the activity. It is important that people with RA learn to listen to their own body and judge the length and type of activity to undertake (ARC, 2007). The podiatrist may also be involved, particularly if the feet are affected, to give advice and help with the assessment of foot function and deformities that affect walking, shoe adaptions, and pain relief.

These potential problems with the activities of daily living require specialist intervention from other members of the multidisciplinary team.

The physiotherapist can assist with exercise and advice regarding activity, rest and the use of joint splints. The occupational therapist can be involved with any adaptions in the home or advise on alternative ways to overcome the problems encountered every day. They can provide utensils to assist with eating and drinking or cooking for the family, for example.

Driving is an activity that can be affected by RA. A car with an automatic gearbox and power steering can assist with hand or foot problems. Other minor adjustments may be necessary, in terms of the seat and position of mirrors. Mobility schemes may be needed for some, or access to high-rate Disability Living Allowance (DLA) with a mobility component (ARC, 2007). The nurse may need to refer their patient to social services for help with this. Other benefits may be accessible as mobility is compromised. Many nurses working in primary care hold their own supply of forms to complete with their client to apply for DLA—this is an important role in tertiary health promotion. There may be a time when the individual requires a wheelchair and these challenges will require support and understanding, as well as resource identification by the nurse and the multidisciplinary team.

## Diet

Anaemia is a common feature of RA, therefore it is important to ensure iron-rich foods are included in addition to a diet that supports the absorption of available dietary iron. The individual may also be prescribed iron supplements. Gaining weight will affect the impact and pain on joints. A healthy balanced diet is all that is required, but the individual may notice flare-ups with certain foods. There is no evidence to support a special diet in RA, although a review by Hagen et al (2009) suggests that there may be some benefit for people who have a Mediterranean or vegetarian diet, but this was not conclusive.

## Emotional health

A person who has RA may feel they will not be able to be involved in their normal social activities, but this should be encouraged and ideas of how this can be achieved should be explored. Friends and family may at first be over-protective and focus on the problem, which can cause anxiety for the patient. Unpredictability may impact on social activity and cause tension in families (ARC, 2007).

Sleep and rest is important to promote cell renewal and protein synthesis. Lack of sleep and rest can have a negative impact on psychological wellbeing and increase pain. Hill and Hale (2004) cited Minor and Westby's

(2001) findings that an individual with an acute inflammatory condition requires 8–10 hours sleep every night in addition 30–60 minutes mid-morning and afternoon. This could be problematic for the parent of a young family, someone who cares for an older relative, or has a demanding job. The nurse will need to discuss the benefits and adaptions that may be necessary to enable this to happen if the patient has a flare-up. Relaxation techniques may help and a member of the multidisciplinary team such as the occupational therapist or physiotherapist may be best placed to teach these techniques.

Intimacy can be problematic for the individual with RA as they experience pain during intercourse and movement may be limited. The nurse should acknowledge this aspect of their patient's life and his/her right to participate in a sexual relationship, despite their chronic health problem. The nurse must feel comfortable and confident to support a person in achieving their goal of continued intimacy in their lives. Booklets may help explain the detail of how to adapt and the nurse should direct the patient to what is available. Other non-statutory agencies may be involved at this point.

---

## Case study 1

*Jane is 48 years old and works fulltime as a housing officer 15 miles from her home. She is married with two children aged 10 and 14 years. Jane's mother has RA and she remembers how, as a child, she and her brothers had to share the household chores after Jane's father left them. Jane has had RA for two years and takes methotrexate with folic acid supplements and sulfasalazine daily. She sometimes forgets one of her tablets and has found this causes flare-ups of her RA.*

- What advice might Jane need from the community nursing team?
- Consider what other members of the multidisciplinary team could offer Jane at this time
- What occupational health issues can you suggest Jane may face?
- Jane will be facing many psychosocial issues in her life. Consider what these might be and how she can be supported with them
- What secondary health promotion advice could the community nurse offer to Jane?

---

---

### Case study 2

*Angela is a 72-year-old widow who has had RA for the last 30 years. She has just been discharged home following arthrodesis to joints in her foot. She lives in a village and likes to participate in all the local social activities.*

- What priorities of care can you identify for Angela using an appropriate nursing model?
- Consider the support individual members of the multidisciplinary team could offer, for example the physiotherapist, occupational therapist, GP, community nurse, social worker, voluntary organizations
- What are the potential pain management issues for Angela?
- Suggest long-term problems that could be experienced by Angela. What health promotion strategies could meet some of these normative and expressed needs?

---

## Conclusion

The King's Fund (2009) found a wide range of quality and service provision across the NHS for people with RA. They also found that health professionals were unaware of the rapid progression of RA. Much of the care they surveyed was based on a medical model of care. In this chapter, a holistic perspective with the patient in the control of their own health journey has been suggested. The King's Fund suggested people with RA receive a 'Cinderella service' unacceptable in our modern health service, especially when the prevalence of this chronic condition is so high. Delay in referral to specialist rheumatology services was mainly as a result of poor knowledge of the effects on the joints in RA.

The nurse can play a vital role in detecting RA, acting as an advocate, promoting independence in the community setting and becoming the key contact to coordinate care provision. The aims of care should focus on symptom relief, maximizing function and reducing the psychological distress and thereby improving the quality of life and empowering the individual with RA (Hill and Hales 2004).

Arnett FC, Edworthy SM, Bloch DA et al (1988) The American Rheumatism Association 1987 revised criteria for the classification of rheumatoid arthritis. *Arthritis Rheum* **31**(3): 315–24

ARC (2006) Rheumatoid Arthritis: An information booklet. http://tinyurl.com/yln64ju (accessed 16 October 2009)

ARC (2007) *Living with Rheumatoid Arthritis.* ARC, London

ARC (2008) Complementary and alternative medicines for the treatment of rheumatoid arthritis, osteoarthritis and fibromyalgia. http://tinyurl.com/yja75dh (accessed 16 October 2009)

ARC (2009) UK arthritis facts—at a glance. http://tinyurl.com/ycr2cll (accessed 16 October 2009)

Blondiaux J, Cotten A, Fontaine C et al (1997) Two Roman and medieval cases of symmetrical erosive polyarthropathy from Normandy: anatomico-pathological and radiological evidence for rheumatoid arthritis. *International Journal of Osteoarchaelogy* 7(5): 451–66

Burbage G (2008) Detecting and managing rheumatoid arthritis. *Pract Nurs* 19(1): 26–30

Combe B, Landewe R, Lukas C et al (2007) EULAR recommendations for the management of early arthritis: report of a task force of the European Standing Committee for International Clinical Studies Including Therapeutics (ESCIST). *Ann Rheum Dis* 66(1): 34–45

DH (2006) The Musculoskeletal Services Framework. DH, London: ref 6857

Edwards SD (1996) *Nursing Ethics: A Principle-based Approach.* Palgrave Macmillan, Basingstoke

Ewles L, Simnett I (2003) *Promoting Health: A Practical Guide.* 5th edn. Scutari, London

Greenstein B, Trounce JR, Gould D (2004) *Trounce's clinical pharmacology for nurses.* 17th edn. Churchill Livingstone, London

Gross R, Kinnison N (2007) *Psychology for Nurses and Allied Health Professionals: Applying Theory to Practice.* Hodder Arnold, London

Hagen KB, Byfuglien MG, Falzon L, Olsen SU, Smedslund G (2009) Dietary interventions for rheumatoid arthritis. *Cochrane Database Syst Rev* (1):CD006400

Hill J, Hale C (2004) Clinical skills: evidence-based nursing care of people with rheumatoid arthritis. *Br J Nurs* 13(14): 852–7

Huizinga TW (2003) Genetics in rheumatoid arthritis. *Best Pract Res Clin Rheumatol* 17(5): 703–16

Joint Formulary Committee (2009) *British National Formulary* 58. September. BMJ Publishing Group Ltd and RPS Publishing, London

Löfman P, Häggman-Laitila A, Pietilä A (2008) Self-determination of patients with rheumatoid arthritis: model development during action research. *Int J Nurs Pract* 14(4): 279–91

Lucas B (2006) *Disorders of the musculoskeletal system.* In: Alexander MF, Fawcett JN, Runciman PJ. eds, *Nursing Practice: Hospital and Home. The Adult.* 3rd edn. Churchill

Livingstone, Edinburgh

Mann EM, Carr E (2009) *Pain: Creative Approaches to Effective Management.* 2nd edn. Palgrave MacMillan, Basingstoke

Melanson PM, Downe-Wamboldt B (2003) Confronting life with rheumatoid arthritis. *J Adv Nurs* **42**(2): 125–33

Minor MA, Westby MR (2001) Rest and exercise. In: Wegener ST. ed, *Clinical Care in the Rheumatic Diseases.* American College of Rheumatology, Atlanta

NAO (2009) Services for people with rheumatoid arthritis. http://tinyurl.com/nsp7fr (accessed 16 October 2009)

NICE (2009) Rheumatoid arthritis. http://guidance.nice.org.uk/CG79 (accessed 16 October 2009)

Niven N (2006) *The Psychology of Nursing Care.* 2nd edn. Palgrave Macmillan, Basingstoke

Nursing and Midwifery Council (2008) *The Code: Standards of conduct, performance and ethics for nurses and midwives.* NMC, London

Nursing Times (2009) New drug may halt progression of rheumatoid arthritis. 16 June. www.nursingtimes.net/5002858.article (accessed 16 October 2009)

Oliver S, Bosworth A, Lax I, Airoldi M (2008) The National Rheumatoid Arthritis Society Mapping Project. http://tinyurl.com/yzogr84 (accessed 9 December 2009)

Orem DE (2001) *Nursing: concepts of practice.* 6th edn. Mosby, St. Louis

Ryan S, Oliver S (2002) Rheumatoid arthritis. Nurs Stand 16(20): 45–52

Symmons D, Turner G, Webb R et al (2002) The prevalence of rheumatoid arthritis in the United Kingdom: new estimates for a new century. *Rheumatology* **41**(7): 793–800

The King's Fund (2009) Perceptions of patients and professionals on rheumatoid arthritis care. http://tinyurl.com/73y7pn (accessed 16 October 2009)

Weiss M, Britten N (2003) What is concordance? *Pharmacy Journal* **271**(7270): 493

# Further reading

Young A (2004) Early Rheumatoid Arthritis Study (ERAS). http://tinyurl.com/yhzkjja (accessed 16 October 2009)

# CHAPTER 7

# Parkinson's disease

*Jean Martey and Jasmin Amoroso*

Parkinson's disease is the second most common cause of chronic neurological disability in the UK (Nutt and Wooten, 2005), and as such, is a significant long-term condition. There are approximately 120 000 people in the UK suffering from Parkinson's disease; on average one person in every 500 is affected by it (Parkinson's Disease Society, 2009a). It affects 8000–10 000 new people in the UK every year (Hotton and Chaudhuri, 2005; NHS Choices, 2007). Future predictions indicate that Parkinson's disease is likely to increase in prevalence in the future due to extension of life expectancy and an ageing population (World Health Organization [WHO], 2006).

Most people are diagnosed between the ages of 50 and 65 years. The risk rises so that by the age of 80 years more than two people per 100 of the population have developed some signs of Parkinson's disease. Young onset disease is identified as those diagnosed below 40 years; this comprises approximately 5% of those diagnosed. There is also a very rare form of the disease, juvenile Parkinson's disease, which affects children (Hotton and Chaudhuri, 2005).

This chapter will present an overview of Parkinson's disease followed by four case studies to illustrate the range of associated issues. Reading this chapter and reflecting on the case studies should enable you to meet the following learning outcomes:

- Identify the characteristics of Parkinson's disease
- Identify some of the challenges in diagnosis
- Identify some of the challenges in the management of Parkinson's disease
- Identify some of the challenges in being a Parkinson's disease sufferer, relative or carer.

## Background

Parkinson's disease is a degenerative neurological disorder of the central nervous system, the cause of which is unknown, although there are many theories. The condition was first identified by Dr James Parkinson (1755–

1824) (Parkinson's Disease Society, 2009b). Research has provided more information about the disease; on a regular basis new features are identified and new medications to treat the symptoms developed. It is known that some symptoms are caused by the death of dopamine-producing cells that lie in the part of the brain called the *substantia nigra*. Depletion of dopamine-producing cells causes reduction in dopamine production (Hotton and Chaudhuri, 2005). Parkinson's disease was the first neurological condition to be linked with a specific chemical deficiency.

In the brain dopamine functions as a chemical messenger that activates dopamine receptors in the striatum, the part of the brain that coordinates movement. As the dopamine-producing cells die, less dopamine is produced and transported to the striatum, making it less able to function normally. Symptoms develop as the neurones die off and dopamine levels drop (Pahwa and Lyons, 2007). Symptoms are characterized as motor and non-motor (Hauser and Zesiewicz, 2006). Motor symptoms include tremor, bradykinesia, rigidity and postural instability (Hauser and Zesiewicz, 2006). Non-motor symptoms are numerous and include: sleep disorders, fatigue, autonomic disturbances, mood and cognitive disorders — patients often report these as more troublesome than motor symptoms (Hauser and Zesiewicz, 2006). Notably, it is not until approximately 80% of these cells have been lost that a reduction in function is noticed. Research suggests that Parkinson's sufferers may also lack other brain chemicals, including serotonin (linked to mood); noradrenaline (linked to blood pressure control); and acetylcholine (linked to mental state) (Hotton and Chaudhuri, 2005).

Parkinson's affects movements such as walking, talking, and writing. However, it is increasingly recognized that Parkinson's is not simply a movement disorder, but is a multisystem neurological disorder which affects cognitive processes, emotion and autonomic function. It can also present as a neuropsychiatric disorder. Up to 33% of those affected progress to developing dementia and 40% develop depression (National Institute for Health and Clinical Excellence [NICE], 2006).

Seriously affected patients may suffer from complications similar to those that occur with many other long-term conditions, for example pneumonia, septicaemia, stroke, urinary tract infection, and pressure sores. Any of these complications can prove to be fatal (Hotton and Chaudhuri, 2005).

## Diagnosis

Parkinson's disease is often difficult to diagnose as patients present in very different ways and as yet, there is no simple test to confirm the diagnosis.

The main three main symptoms of the disease and those that are used in the diagnosis are tremor, bradykinesia and rigidity (NICE, 2006). Tremor (shaking) is usually noticed in one limb when a person is relaxed; it stops on movement then returns again on rest—it can increase with anxiety or excitement. This is known a pill-rolling tremor (only 70% of people with Parkinson's will have a tremor) (Pahwa and Lyons, 2007). Bradykinesia (slowness) is usually seen as a general slowing down, but can affect fine movement and coordination Rigidity (stiffness) has two types: 'lead pipe rigidity', where the limb shows a resistance on repetitive movement; and 'cogwheel rigidity', where smooth movement is replaced with a ratchet-type movement normally felt in the wrist and elbow joints. This leads to problems with mobility and non-verbal communication, and can be painful.

However, Parkinson's disease can cause many other symptoms:

- Poor balance and unstable walking (shuffling, difficulty in turning, falls)
- Inability to concentrate
- Depression and anxiety
- Frozen shoulder
- General slowing down/lethargy
- Clumsiness
- Dragging a leg/arm
- Expressionless face
- Speech and swallowing problems
- Reduced manual dexterity, including handwriting difficulties
- Drooling
- Constipation
- Sleep problems
- Urination at night (nocturia)
- Difficulty in turning in bed at night.

Diagnosis is primarily clinical, based on history and examination (NICE, 2006). For a patient to be diagnosed with Parkinson's disease, he/she must present with two of the three main symptoms, although it may take many years for this to happen, leading to frustration and anguish for suffers and their families. At first, minor difficulties begin to surface, though these may still appear unrelated to Parkinson's disease, such as constipation, lethargy or painful shoulders. Furthermore, features such as a general slowing down, having difficulty getting up out of a low chair, problems turning in bed, and not able to keep up with the crowd, may be wrongly attributed to the ageing process.

The disease will continue to progress, and prompt, accurate clinical diagnosis is important; people with suspected Parkinson's should be referred quickly and untreated to a specialist (NICE, 2006). However, it is often not until someone identifies that the symptoms have a possible link to a more serious condition, that a referral is made to a specialist. Therefore, it may take a number of years for a formal diagnosis to be made.

Diagnosis is confirmed through response to medication; however, there are a number of conditions that mimic Parkinson's disease. These might initially respond, albeit in minor way, to medication, but after few years the response dwindles and the disease progression escalates. These people are then classed as having 'Parkinsonisms' and are still cared for by the same specialist neurology teams.

## Treatment

In theory, it would be useful to replace dopamine through medical therapy. However, dopamine does not cross the blood–brain barrier, so administration is of no use. The first breakthrough in treatment was the development of levodopa in the 1960s, which is the single most effective anti-Parkinson treatment. Levodopa is converted into dopamine in the brain by an enzyme, dopa decarboxylase (DDC); this led to the development of Sinemet and Madopar. These enable replacement of depleted dopamine production, which leads to an improvement of symptoms.

Levodopa remains the gold-standard therapy. Most patients notice an improvement almost immediately, although some may not for many months or years. Short-term side-effects are uncommon, but include nausea, hallucinations, tiredness and light-headedness. However, virtually all patients suffer long-term complications. Approximately 50–75% of those taking the drug for 5–10 years develop abnormally excessive and involuntary movements called dyskinesias (Hotton and Chaudhuri, 2005).

Since the introduction of levodopa, new therapies have been developed. In the 1960s dopamine agonists were developed, which were introduced in the mid 1970s. These work by directly stimulating the dopamine receptors to bypass the degenerating brain cells. They are less effective than levodopa in advanced disease, but clinically indicated in early untreated Parkinson's. Treatment with dopamine agonists reduces the chance of dyskinesias by up to 50% (Parkinson's Disease Society, 2009a). This shows that it is beneficial to start treatment with dopamine agonists in younger patients, and therefore delay the requirement for levodopa (Hotton and Chaudhuri, 2005).

The side-effects of dopamine agonists are similar to levodopa, but nausea and hallucinations usually occur more often. Patients are commonly prescribed an antiemetic for at least the first two weeks of treatment

(Hotton and Chaudhuri, 2005). Since 2005, reports have emerged that some people taking dopamine agonists demonstrate odd side-effects, for example patients becoming compulsive gamblers, when they never previously gambled, and some complaining of a compulsive desire for sex, with sexual behaviours that were not normal for them (Dodd et al, 2005). Overeating, overspending and other compulsions can occur (Nirenberg and Waters, 2006). These behaviours were reported to cause sufferers, relatives and carers considerable distress.

More recently, attention has been paid to the prevention of the breakdown of dopamine. It is recognized that substances which occur naturally in the body cause the breakdown of dopamine (European Parkinson's Disease Association [EPDA], 2008), for example DDC, catechol-O-methyl transferase (COMT) and monoamine oxidase B (MAOB) (EPDA, 2008). Therapies now aim at the prevention of dopamine breakdown, which enables dopamine to reach higher levels in the brain and survive longer— with an enhanced therapeutic effect.

Brain surgery, to structures deep within the brain known as the subthalamic nucleus, the globus pallidus and the thalamus, can be offered. These have been shown to reduce symptoms in some patients (NICE, 2006). Operations may involve lesioning (destroying cells in a target area by burning a hole); however, most operations today involve deep stimulation— electrically stimulating cells using a pacemaker or transplantation.

Notably, all treatments treat the symptoms of Parkinson's disease, but do not treat the disease itself. Once a diagnosis has been made, then the decision is made of whether to treat or whether watchful waiting is appropriate.

There are a variety of theories on when to treat, but none offer robust supporting evidence (Lees, 2009). Immediate treatment is thought by some to be neuro-protective, but there is no evidence to support this (Lees, 2009). Alternatively, NICE (2006) recommends pharmacotherapy once motor symptoms begin to impair the patient's functional ability. Long-term use of all drugs for the treatment of symptoms can have adverse effects, increasing sufferers' disabilities (Lang, 2009). Therefore, treatment should involve an informed decision made by the patient Once the decision to treat is made, the treatment modality should be decided, based on the symptoms, age and disability of the patient. There is no single drug of choice in the initial treatment of early Parkinson's disease. The choice of drug first prescribed should take into account clinical and lifestyle characteristics and patient preference, after the patient has been informed of the short- and long-term benefits and drawbacks of each type of medication. First choice pharmacological therapy options include levodopa, dopamine agonists, and MAOB inhibitors (NICE, 2006).

# Case studies

Four case studies are now presented. The cases were co-managed by the medical team and a Parkinson's disease nurse specialist. The role of the specialist nurse involves providing clinical, psychological and social support for patients and their families. The nurse is an advisor who has specialist knowledge, and an educator to all. Often, this nurse is the only constant member of the healthcare team that a patient gets to know. Many patients are seen by different registrars or GPs at each visit to either hospital or their general practice. As a result, patients often confide in the nurse more openly than the doctor; they appear to be seen as more accessible, despite having large caseloads.

Parkinson's disease nurse specialists work in conjunction with the medical team and also work autonomously. This includes running nurse-led clinics in both hospital and community settings, seeing people within their own homes, and visiting them in hospital where necessary. Every nurse works differently, but within NICE (2006) guidelines, which advocate that these nurses:

- Monitor and adjust medication
- Act as a point of contact for support and if necessary offer home visits
- Provide reliable information regarding clinical and social matters to both patients and their carers.

Some nurses are based in secondary care and others in primary care settings. However, all work towards the common aim of providing patients with Parkinson's disease with the best locally-available care

Analysis of the case studies will give you the opportunity to consider these factors through real-life examples and to identify the key points that you have learned.

## Case study 1

Jane is aged 34 years and married with three boys aged 6, 8 and 10 years. She initially presented with worsening stiffness, inability to coordinate and painful spasms. Her past medical history included depression and obsessive behaviour. At first she was suspected of suffering from dystonia; a condition often seen in young women, causing severe muscle spasms, plus possible psychological components. Twelve months of extensive tests and a positive response to medication produced a working diagnosis of Parkinson's disease. Jane was initially started on ropinirole, a non-ergot dopamine agonist and one of the firstline therapies used in young-onset Parkinson's disease. The rationale was that she had many years of medication in front of her, so levodopa, which has many side-effects, should be reserved for later.

Jane responded well initially, but her dose soon increased to the maximum. After a few months, her control began to fluctuate and medication doses lasted for shorter periods. When the medication worked she had good mobility and control enabling her to lead a normal life, taking the children to school, walking the dogs, and managing the household chores. Once the medication began to lose its effect and fluctuate, this control was lost. At times the medication would be effective, and at other times it had no effect; then she had very little mobility and severe pain.

This left Jane with increasing difficulties coping as a young mother. It is preferable to manage young patients on a regimen that does not include levodopa for as long as possible. In this case it was impossible; levodopa was added less than one year after diagnosis. The concern when using levodopa is that side-effects will quickly follow, causing involuntary movements (dyskinesia) which can be as disabling as the disease. Dyskinesia became evident within a few months.

A COMT inhibitor was added to improve absorption and thereby increase the amount of levodopa in Jane's system, without increasing the amount of levodopa that she needed to take. This increased mobility and improved control. Three years post-diagnosis, Jane is already on triple therapy and taking medication every three hours. What the future holds is not known, as there is no set pattern for Parkinson's disease. It is important to watch and wait and see how the disease progresses, treating each symptom as it arises.

---

### Reflection

Reflect on what you have learned about Parkinson's disease from case study 1. Did you note the following:

- Parkinson's can occur at a young age
- Parkinson's would not be the first differential diagnosis in such cases; alternatives would be investigated, thereby delaying diagnosis
- Treatment might be required following diagnosis, but treatments can lose their beneficial effect quickly and can cause disabling side-effects
- Levodopa is deferred for as long as possible owing to severe side-effects
- It is likely that multiple therapy will be required as the condition progresses
- Treatment will be based on minimizing symptoms *and* minimizing side-effects
- Treatment must involve consideration of benefit *versus* harm.

## Case study 2

Fred is a 69-year-old retired managing director of a large company. He has travelled the world, living outside the UK for many years. Taking early retirement at 55 years, his plan was to build his own house, play golf and go to lunch with is old work colleagues, while his wife continued her voluntary work at a local hospice. His diagnosis at the age of 63 years came as a shock. He had noticed a slight tremor in his right hand along with a stiffness in his shoulder. Initially, it was thought that this was an injury related to playing golf, but after a course of physiotherapy, with no improvement to the tremor and little improvement to function, he was referred to a neurology specialist for an opinion.

Treatment was initiated following diagnosis. The tremor was treated with benzhexol, which has subsequently been exchanged for tryhexiphenidyl. Stiffness was treated with the dopamine agonist pramipexole. Four years later, levodopa was added when control began to fluctuate. The fluctuations brought dystonic spasms which affected his mobility. Medication was increased and fractionated, so that he took medication on a two-hourly basis.

After seven years of managing on oral medication, Fred was referred for insertion of deep brain stimulators, which are inserted into the subthalamic nucleus. Deep brain stimulation (DBS) controls the symptoms of Parkinson's disease by altering the electrical circuitry of the mid-brain, enabling oral medication to be reduced, and in some cases removed completely. The use of DBS in late-stage Parkinson's replaces the effect or adds to the effect of medication improving control.

Depression can be a side-effect of DBS insertion and unfortunately, Fred became extremely depressed. He was treated with a course of selective serotonin reuptake inhibitors (SSRIs) and counselling. Fred will probably need to remain on some form of anti-depressant for the rest of his life. Although the surgery has been a success in reducing some of the symptoms of Parkinson's disease, his control is not perfect.

Many patients find this difficult to accept following surgery, as expectations can be high and managing the disappointment can be difficult and response to medication is also reduced both physically and psychologically.

Many patients who have undergone surgery will return to a relatively high level of medication following surgery in a bid to regain the 'buzz' effect they received from their medication before surgery. Getting the dose right can be difficult and too much medication can cause an increase in symptoms, causing distress.

---

**Reflection**

Reflect on what you have learned about Parkinson's disease from case study 2. Did you note the following:
- Parkinson's is not always the first differential diagnosis; alternatives might be investigated, thereby delaying diagnosis
- Treatment might be required following diagnosis, but treatments can lose their beneficial effects
- It is likely that multiple therapy will be required as the condition progresses
- Levodopa is deferred for as long as possible owing to severe side-effects
- Surgery is an adjunctive treatment for Parkinson's disease; however, it is not curative and can cause additional problems as well as being beneficial
- Depression can occur as a severe side-effect of surgery
- Expectations of surgery can be unrealistically high, and even when benefits are evident, disappointment can be severe
- Careful counselling is required both before and after surgery.

---

## Case study 3

Geoffrey is 79 years old. His symptoms include slowness, stooped posture, slight tremor in his left hand, and constipation. He was diagnosed with Parkinson's disease. Slowly, over the past five years, he had become increasing disabled. He now finds it difficult to dress himself, using the bath is impossible, and his wife is helping him with a strip-wash every day; she is also 79 years old, but in good health.

As a result of his poor posture, Geoffrey's mobility was reduced, he tired easily, his voice had become quiet (though he blamed his wife's hearing), and he had occasionally choked on his food—this had been linked to ill-fitting dentures. During the past six months, he had increasingly withdrawn from conversation and slept many days away.

Taking his increasing disability into account, it was decided to initiate therapy using levodopa three times daily. Over the next few weeks, his symptoms slowly improved. With the help of physiotherapy and occupational therapy, his mobility and ability to function independently improved to the point that he was convinced he did not have the disease, then suddenly his symptoms increased and he became confused, with hallucinations. His symptoms escalated so quickly that the GP had him admitted to hospital. Geoffrey was diagnosed with a urinary tract infection and treated with antibiotics. However, his confusion escalated and he refused his medication. Over the next few weeks, the psychiatric team became involved and antipsychotic medication was initiated. Things slowly began to improve; his mobility improved to the point he could walk with a zimmer frame, and his confusion improved, although he still had the occasional hallucination. Social services were mobilized and a care package was set up to enable his discharge. Unfortunately he never completely recovered.

Many patients are admitted to hospital with infections causing a sudden deterioration in their condition. Whenever possible, medication regimens should remain as they were before admission and the infection treated. If this is not possible, then advice should ideally be sought from the consultant who manages the patient's condition—stopping medication suddenly can result in neuroleptic malignant syndrome, which can be fatal.

Many patients are taking medication that does not fit neatly into a ward drug round; it is important to try to keep the timing of medication stable and all effort should be made to maintain a patient's regular regimen as changes can alter control and take months to correct.

---

**Reflection**

Reflect on what you have learned about Parkinson's disease from case study 3. Did you note the following:
- Parkinson's is not always the first differential diagnosis; alternatives might be investigated, thereby delaying diagnosis
- Physiotherapy and occupational therapy can be very useful in the management of Parkinson's disease
- When suffering from Parkinson's, like any other long-term condition, acute complications can occur and infections are common
- Treatment for other conditions, such as infections, should not exclude treatment for Parkinson's
- Cessation of treatment for Parkinson's should not occur despite other acute conditions requiring treatment
- Specialist advice might be required when managing a Parkinson's patient who requires care for an acute complication.

## Case study 4

John is 69 years old and married for a second time to a woman 20 years his junior and who works full-time. They have an eight-year-old child. John has two children in their 30s from his first marriage. He was diagnosed three years ago, with rigidity and bradykinesia but no tremor. John took early retirement at the age of 60 years, is a stay-at-home dad and looks after his elder daughter's two horses, mucking out and exercising them daily, and managing the paddock.

John sold his business for a good profit and has no money worries. He likes to gamble at the casino occasionally, but limits himself to £150 per visit. He enjoys socializing, has a good group of younger active friends and until now, has been able to keep up. On diagnosis John commenced a dopamine agonist, Mirapexin 1.5 mg twice daily. This is a high dose as the British National Formulary (Joint Formulary Committee, 2009) recommends 'initially 88 µ three times daily, dose doubled every 5–7 days if tolerated to 350 µ three times daily; further increased if necessary by 180 µ three times daily at weekly intervals'. The maximum dosage is 3.3 mg daily in three divided doses. However, John's consultant prescribed in accordance with John's stated need to be normal and not show any signs of the disease. (Consultants have the clinical freedom to prescribe outside of clinical guidelines.)

For the past two months his wife has noticed a change in his personality; John has become more demanding in the bedroom, more argumentative, and wanting to go out to the casino at unusual times. This was always something they did as a couple, whereas now he insists on going alone. One weekend he spent in excess of £2000, which caused a huge argument and John's wife vented her suspicions of his having an affair. At this point, John broke down and admitted to a gambling compulsion that he couldn't control; he assured her that he was not seeing another woman.

An emergency appointment with Parkinson's disease nurse specialist was made. John admitted to losing in excess of £10 000 over a two-month period, and to having an increasing urge for sexual gratification, which was becoming so bad he had considered going outside of the marriage, but as yet had not.

His medication was immediately reduced, with further reduction planned; it would eventually be removed and replaced with levodopa. An appointment was made through their GP for counselling, and both husband and wife were initiated on antidepressants to help them cope. Two months later, the gambling had returned to a social outing for them both, their sex life, though not yet back to normal, is improving. His mobility, however, is now a little compromised. He will now be stabilized on levodopa preparations, with adjunct therapy to increase its absorption.

---

**Reflection**

Reflect on what you have learned about Parkinson's disease from case study 4. Did you note the following:

*   The symptoms of Parkinson's can be profoundly embarrassing for a sufferer
*   Mirapexin (indeed, all dopamine agonists) can cause significant side-effects, such as compulsive gambling, extreme sexual behaviours, overeating, overspending and other compulsions
*   The treatment of Parkinson's can cause marital or other relationship difficulties
*   Concordance is essential, especially engendering the trust of patients relatives and carers about side-effects
*   Counselling may be required.

---

## Conclusion

This chapter has described Parkinson's disease and outlined the levels of incidence. The challenges of diagnosis and management have been discussed. These challenges were illustrated using four case studies, which showed the difficulties in making a diagnosis and how this can be delayed through consideration of differential factors associated with being young or growing old. The case studies also showed that success of medical therapies may be both variable and short lived; furthermore, medical therapies commonly cause distressing side-effects that have a profound impact on sufferers, relatives and carers.

Dodd ML, Klos KJ, Bower JH, Geda YE, Josephs KA, Ahlskog JE (2005) Pathological gambling caused by drugs used to treat Parkinson disease. *Arch Neurol* **62**(9): 1377–81

European Parkinson's Disease Association (2008) Drug treatment options. http://tinyurl.com/yzeoqtz (accessed 10 December 2009)

Hauser R, Zesiewicz TA (2006) *Parkinson's Disease: Questions and Answers.* Merit Publishing International, Surrey

Hotton G, Chaudhuri R (2005) Parkinson's disease. http://tinyurl.com/yl45ycc (accessed 23 October 2009)

Joint Formulary Committee (2009) *British National Formulary* 58. September. BMJ Publishing Group Ltd and RPS Publishing, London

Lang A (2009) When and how should treatment be started in Parkinson's disease? *Neurology* **72**: 39–43

Lees A (2009) Parkinson's disease therapy—when to start and what to choose. *Eur Neurol* **3**(2): 34–6

NHS Choices (2007) Parkinson's disease. www.nhs.uk/Conditions/Parkinsons-disease (accessed 10 December 2009)

NICE (2006) Parkinson's disease: diagnosis and management in primary and secondary care. http://guidance.nice.org.uk/CG35 (accessed 23 October 2009)

Nirenberg M, Waters C (2006) Compulsive eating and weight gain related to dopamine agonist use. *Mov Disord* **21**(4): 524–9

Nutt JG, Wooten GF (2005) Diagnosis and initial management of Parkinson's disease. *New Engl J Med* **353**: 1021–7

Pahwa R, Lyons K (2007) *Handbook of Parkinson's Disease*. Informa Healthcare, USA

Parkinson's Disease Society (2009a) The Professional's Guide to Parkinson's Disease http://tinyurl.com/yfow4ou (accessed 10 December 2009)

Parkinson's Disease Society (2009b) About Parkinson's. http://tinyurl.com/yjowm9d (accessed on 23 October 2009)

WHO (2006) Neurological Disorders. Public Health Challenges. http://tinyurl.com/64anp7 (accessed 10 December 2009)

# CHAPTER 8

# Living with a frayed brain: a patient perspective

*Tony Robinson*

*The following account is given by Tony, a former youth worker aged 54 years, who has lived with Parkinson's disease for over 10 years. Tony has a background in education and a partner who works in the health service. His account aims to explain the impact of diagnosis and the realities of living with a neurological condition. His exploration through personal experience illustrates the increasing pressures that have influenced all aspects of his life as a result of this condition. He highlights some of the major challenges he has encountered and describes some of the coping mechanisms that he has developed to enable him to meet these challenges.*

> Parkinson's disease is a progressive neurological condition. It occurs as a result of a loss of nerve cells in the part of the brain known as the *substantia nigra*. These cells are responsible for producing dopamine, a chemical which allows messages to be sent to the parts of the brain that coordinate movement.

One of the perils of listening to a person with Parkinson's is that you (the professional) become detached or bored after the first half hour of descriptive monologue, with which you struggle to find rapport/empathy. The challenge, on the other hand, is that you are obliged to extrapolate from that welter of difficult information a clinical analysis or insight that will, in turn, inform your understanding and ultimately attune your empathy. When you then interject the extreme variations in the patient's symptoms and reactions to treatment (e.g. one person's 'ideal drug' is another's nightmare hallucinatory experience), you could rapidly come to the conclusion that the condition is either despairingly complex, or something bordering on what the media portray as a 'designer illness'.

What does the individual do to cope with this? In one of his books, the American author Bill Bryson poses an open and unanswered question: Why on earth do people flock with such enthusiasm to the Parkinson's convention? My reply, and that I believe of most Parkinson's sufferers, would be obvious: to share and collectively understand our medical condition and to thereby gain self-affirmation—that rarely acknowledged aspect of good mental health in 'ordinary' human beings. Such networking, whether through a convention or the more modern tool of the internet, is of particular importance in an illness where symptoms, drug reactions and methods of coping are so widely variable from one individual to another, and where isolation can expose you to the danger of depression and other forms of psychological stress.

In order to bridge the gap between the two worlds described in the first two paragraphs, I will occasionally attempt to find examples of descriptive metaphor or partial parallels to 'ordinarily experienced life' to bring the Parkinson's agenda to the uninitiated. I also will occasionally refer to symptoms and situations described to me by other people with Parkinson's, but not experienced myself.

## Diagnosis

Every one of us arrives at an illness equipped with our individual set of emotional, social and intellectual templates, and our personality will help dictate how we cope. To give an example of extremes, intellectual knowledge may help one person cope better with an illness, whereas it may lead another into the realms of deepest despair and pessimism. Parkinson's disease, with its multifaceted array of symptoms, can normally guarantee to find you out—if you find yourself coping well with one aspect of the illness, another aspect will knock you off your feet. Diagnosis and your reaction to it can be a key area of professional intervention, in my opinion. It may be assumed by the professional that shock and denial will be common early symptoms, and, speaking to those who were quickly diagnosed, I would agree. However, I found myself among a sizeable cohort of patients who struggle for years to get a diagnosis, in which case your mind is infused for some time with a cloud of conflicting emotion—a sense of relief (Parkinson's in itself is not life-threatening) mixed with bewildered anger. To keep my diagnostic description brief, I will simply list some points without elaborating too much on my three-year wait:

- If a patient crosses the surgery doors with a whole list of unusual symptoms and has barely even 'called in' during the previous 10 years on the books, do not immediately assume that he/she is a hypochondriac

- Do not start questions exclusively with 'where does it hurt?' The patient who keeps insisting that, for no explicable reason, 'one of my legs does not work properly and this leads to pains in my knees', may merit neurological as well as orthopaedic enquiry
- When the above is accompanied with a blank facial expression please add it to your 'possibly neurological' list, rather than assume a separate diagnosis of depression (admittedly, depression can be an accompaniment to the illness)
- Most importantly, if your sole diagnostic template for Parkinson's is that of bilateral tremor in the elderly, update your skills. Younger people do suffer from the condition in statistically significant numbers, and three out of ten Parkinson's patients present on diagnosis with irregular, stiff and slow limb movement and no tremor.

## Impact on lifestyle and occupation

This is an area with which I recall having severe discomfort in the initial years of diagnosis, but which I can now view with a greater degree of equanimity. Obviously, certain situations contribute to this—holding onto a job is different to being retired, for example. However, there is a perspective with a degenerative condition that is unavoidable; that of falling from the great height of 'normal function' to undefined depths of dysfunction. I once compared it to the vision of yourself as a skydiver having just left the plane, finding that your main chute has failed and struggling to get your reserve chute to work. Most of the help that is offered seems to be located on the ground, when what you immediately need is a more experienced skydiver to help you with that stubborn reserve chute, or to rescue you in some improbably heroic manner. I would see the early stage after diagnosis as the time which merits most input of psychological support and help with adaption.

Have you ever experienced sharing a kitchen area with someone staggering around with a hangover, or severely slowed by some illness or injury? In those instances how often have you said, 'for goodness sake get back to bed or sit on the sofa for a while, I am trying to get ready for work'. To varying degrees, this can happen every single day. In our own domestic situation, this 'slowing down phenomenon' combined with my diminished ability to rapidly adjust limb movement, and meant that one day I ended up jammed shoulder-to-shoulder in the front door frame with my partner. Humorous to recall now, but a cause of argument at the time (worsened by the non-diagnosed status of my illness).

Another aspect of Parkinson's disease that intrudes into your life is a slowing down or lack of facial expression or body language. This intrudes first and foremost into your relationships with family or friends. 'You aren't listening, are you?' can be a prime opening line in any argument. There is the training exercise sometimes used in youth work when one person acts as a listener while their partner talks about something that would normally be of mutual interest. The 'listener' is briefed to turn away their body or avert their eyes while offering verbally positive but unemphatic affirmation or agreement. I can vouch for the fact that if you are the one 'being listened to', you want to hit your so-called 'listener' after a while, even if you are not usually moved to violence. Such can be the social implications of some Parkinson's symptoms.

What about the work implications for a person with Parkinson's? Every work perspective is different, but I would suggest that work requiring repeated manual dexterity or strength will soon find you out and make it very difficult for you to continue. I base this on experience that putting up a single shelf can extend from taking a normal half hour into a Parkinson's half-day. But what about a job that requires less manually-focused skills? Many organizations, such as the one I worked for, are willing to go to considerable lengths to accommodate you. However, even the best incremental assessment of disability impact can prove ineffective in taking on board the variable nature of a condition such as Parkinson's disease.

I will approach the list of typically difficult work tasks from what would seem to be an oblique angle, but what I hope will be another translatable parallel to ordinary experience. Books written about Parkinson's disease often mention the adverse effects of stress on the condition. Typically, the effects vary from individual to individual, but people do run their lives and jobs on varying degrees of stress and adrenalin. In extreme instances of stress, ordinary people can be 'frozen in fear', 'lost for words', or left 'feeling numb and drained of energy'. Some of us even choose a challenging job (or life) that requires a careful coordination and harnessing of adrenalin, which, if you are successful, is rewarded in your nervous system by the release of a copious amount of dopamine. When I admit to having had a long-term commitment to rock climbing, and to career choices in special needs (emotional/behavioural disturbance) and youth work (both challenging and variable people-based jobs), you probably have an inkling of how I like my dopamine served up, and some inkling of how it would impact on my life. What would seem to happen (this is, clinically, a layman's speculation) is that adrenalin kicks in against your initial stream of depleted dopamine. The upshot can be that you are reduced to tremor or stiff lethargy just when you need to act, or perhaps just after you have acted.

I will give two stark examples of this in my life. In the year before my wandering leg symptom, I was on a school caving trip demonstrating how to do a not too challenging squeeze through a short rock tunnel, when my body suddenly refused to wriggle and the leader of the group spent at least 20 minutes coaxing and advising alternatives to wriggling before successfully getting me out. It was not the best time to experience your first noticeable symptom. Another example came shortly before I gave up work. I rashly volunteered to pursue a couple of rebellious older youths who were set on provoking pupils and staff throughout the school site. Using the best of my skills and my existing relationship with them in less confrontational situations, I got them to leave the site of their own volition before the police arrived. I went back up to the headteacher's office to what should have been a congratulatory chat and temporary 'adrenalin break', at which point my limbs froze almost completely and I could barely put together two consecutive words. These examples are extreme instances of adrenalin use, but lesser inputs of adrenalin structure our lives. Unfulfilled use of adrenalin, such as when you're running late and get stuck in a traffic jam, or when a series of unscheduled events foil your plans at work, can induce headaches and other physical symptoms. With Parkinson's, the physical symptoms can become much worse. You become vulnerable to stress in a way that would be deemed by 'ordinary people' as 'unusual'. Inside you may still retain sustaining self-confidence, but this becomes increasingly difficult to display (and, importantly, to reward yourself for).

At which point did I retire? When a 'good day' consisted of having arrived at work free of any domestic stress or travel frustration; when 'bad news' or problems are kept from you until later; when you didn't get angry with yourself for taking 10 minutes selecting three bits of paper from a filing cabinet for a meeting; when the meeting went smoothly and without a need for argument; and when the fatigue that plagues you did not reduce you to a 20 minute 'power nap' until later in the afternoon. My employer was willing to go on accommodating my disability. I was not.

I must add that this is my personal experience of how adrenalin impacts—a conversation with an expert from the Parkinson's Disease Society reminded me that another cohort of Parkinson's disease sufferers can effectively only 'get themselves going' if they spur themselves on by engagement in adrenalin-inducing activities.

## Methods of coping

You may have surmised that adaption is a key strategy for coping with Parkinson's disease. Everyone has their own strategy and there is a complex area of overlap between adaption, acceptance and the determination to fight on. Personality comes into play and arguments can occur. One person's adaption strategy may, in their own opinion, be a good example of being determined and fighting on. Someone else may hear of it and think (or even say), 'if I did that, I would just be giving in and succumbing to the condition'. As Parkinson's disease is a progressive condition, this kind of debate between defeatism and adaption is recurrent. An image comes to mind of the reaction of sunbathers on a beach to an incoming tide. Some choose to adapt by small degrees every five minutes, taking on board the attendant risks of being given a soaking by a sudden surge of seawater. Others, on spotting the turning tide, retreat to a respectable distance from the incoming waves (and that can vary from 20 feet to the point last achieved by a high-tide in a record year). Most of us set our towels at a range of points during different stages on that Parkinson's beach, even when facing different combinations of symptoms. I will give you an example where I have adopted my own method of coping (I can assure you, there are many others).

Shopping can be a thing we either love or loathe, but, whatever your feelings, most of us experience it. Grocery shopping has never been a popular part of my weekly schedule, but since I developed Parkinson's, it has presented a new range of challenges. The first is the dilemma of whether or not to identify yourself as disabled. Carrying a walking stick in your trolley may be superfluous to need and can actually be a disadvantage when you try to retrieve it while fumbling with goods, cards/money/receipts, and till small-talk (multitasking is a common crisis point for most Parkinson's sufferers); however, it does stop you from being identified as a 'fraudulent' member of the disabled community, as you stumble out of your car in the disabled bay and in usual Parkinson's haste head for the nearest trolley for physical support. The other contact is with the supermarket staff. My earlier set of Parkinson's symptoms (when I could get around to and from a trolley instead of making it an item of physical support) included staggering from side to side, a blank facial expression, and taking an unusual amount of time checking the price or ingredients on tins. These symptoms are very similar to those that supermarket staff are asked by management to follow closely as the likely outcome is that you are dealing with an alcohol-fuelled potential shoplifter. After a very close experience of being followed step-by-step around a local supermarket, I fired off an angry disability-awareness letter to supermarket HQ that the youth worker in me felt entitled to deliver. The reply admitted no responsibility (i.e. it could be just a subjective over-reaction to ordinary levels of supermarket vigilance), and they could arrange for a 'clear the air' meeting with their stalwart local supermarket manager. To fully empathize with this new dilemma, I must refer to an earlier described symptom of finding myself lost for words when undergoing adrenalin-inducing episodes in my life. I could envisage myself speechless, but raging inside before this urbane supermarket manager, who, between his bland and unchallenged reassurances, would be feeling smugly vindicated in his assessment of me as a rather enfeebled member of the public overreacting as a result of the awful condition from which I suffered. I simply wrote a letter saying I would not be shopping there anymore.

## Relationships with services and agencies

Incapacity assessment is an area of current controversy for all disabled people and normally elicits a visceral response. The Government aspires to a new notion that disabled people should be assessed according to what they can do, rather than what they cannot (offering certain limited incentives if you choose to move in their defined direction). Yet, the main tool of the Department of Work and Pensions and other agencies is an incremental assessment of certain set tasks that reward you financially when you prove what you cannot do, using their exacting criteria (which normally extends to 20 pages of repetitive and not always relevant questions in three separate booklets). If your assessment is subsequently questioned in some way, your ordeal will be highlighted in the local press and there will be one thing that is assured; neither the press nor agency pursuing the case will give any credence to the idea that the system of assessment is at fault. The press will label you as a scrounger, deserving of heinous punishment, and the agency will list you as a person who has 'wrongly presented the facts', or has failed to inform them of 'an improvement in your condition'.

A few aspects of this procedure particularly impact on the Parkinson's applicant:

- Having a progressively degenerative condition, you will probably need to fill in the same forms at different points of your illness (and you will be reminded that you risk losing your existing lower-level benefit when being assessed for a higher level)
- Parkinson's disease is a bizarre disability. It is not unusual for someone to have difficulty walking, yet maintain the ability to run or do a set of martial arts moves. I myself can walk backwards or hop with moderate success, yet constantly struggle to walk forward. There seems to be a 'relic survival' in the brain of a certain degree of coordination and this can sometimes be enhanced by timely dosages of medication or sequences of movement or exercise. Try getting that down onto a form which insists that your condition must progress in pleasingly systematic, incremental stages, and which does not even offer 'lack of coordination' as a reason for 'not walking' or 'falling over' for example
- Incremental assessment does not lend itself to the daily ups and downs of a variable condition like Parkinson's. You can imagine the telephone

query answers: 'On a good day I can walk 200 yards, on a bad day I can't walk at all, and on the days in between...'. 'What percentage of good days do you have?' asks the exasperated official on the end of the phone. You return with your calculator 10 minutes later.

## Nursing implications?

The following section is based on my personal surmising about some of the situations the Parkinson's patient may encounter on a nursing ward. I assume a greater depth of knowledge from my anticipated readers, hence the use of a question-mark in the heading.

To put Parkinson's in the context of a ward, where staff are, primarily, more focused on incremental progression (e.g. recovery from a broken limb), the condition must sit in the chronic illness category, where the pathway through the clinical goals of care, medical intervention and recovery are made more complicated, if not compromised, by the underlying and persisting condition. It is even possible that the progress to 'successful' acute recovery may be accompanied by a worsening of other symptoms of mental health or dysfunction. When you then throw in for good measure the current tendency of the Government to bring in so many simultaneous initiatives that every member of staff at the coal-face is operating on capacity overload, I can understand if the welcoming smile of the ward nurse is somewhat strained.

I recently read a book called *Mind*, in which the author ambitiously attempts to define how the mind works, and uses the malfunctioning brain as a reference point, or as a leading element in his scientific argument (e.g. because the damaged or malfunctioning brain presents as x, the healthy brain's function must be y). The author suggests a reference to the 'frayed' brain to describe categories of deteriorating function, such as Parkinson's disease. I would like to borrow and develop this image, as a useful tool in describing the Parkinson's disease process and how best to apply the concept of 'fraying' in its original context of fabric, an accompanying recollection of darning comes to mind. One way of viewing the needs of a Parkinson's patient would be to envisage their daily mental dysfunctions in terms of a number of different areas of 'fraying', which can be partly 'darned' or repaired by introducing a daily variety of social, physical or medicinal inputs.

Whether or not this image works for you, I would like to end by offering some useful reminders or possible questions to consider in a nursing context:

- Have you read the relevant leaflets on Parkinson's disease, such as 'Get it on time', and accessed information from a Parkinson's disease nurse specialist or other relevant professional?
- Have you talked directly to the patient and/or a knowledgeable carer?
- Have you familiarized yourself with possible Parkinson's disease symptoms that may be confused with acute symptoms for concern (a sudden seizing up, for example)?
- Do you have any flexibility on your ward or area? If a person functions far better physically in the mornings and physiotherapy sessions are scheduled for afternoons, can any adaptions be made to this routine? It may lead to a speedier recovery.

*It is evident from Tony's account that the challenges of living with a long-term condition impact on every aspect of daily life. It is interesting to note that the patient experience often begins well in advance of diagnosis, a period in which patients may encounter some degree of worrying and life-altering symptoms. Subsequent diagnosis is not always straightforward and may, for some patients, be a prolonged and stressful process. The quality of the patient experience at this time underpins the development of an effective therapeutic relationship. The consequences of which may influence subsequent relationships and confidence in health professionals.*

*Tony's account raises some interesting points for consideration from a nursing perspective; the importance of developing effective communication skills and the ability to use an empathetic approach that also respects the individuality and uniqueness of each patient journey. It is important that we recognize that quality of life is specific to each individual, and this emphasizes the importance of adopting a holistic approach and personalized care plan.*

---

### Reflection

- What are the most important quality of life issues for Tony?
- You might like to read this chapter in conjunction with the next chapter, which explores the experiences of a carer
- Are there any parallels or similarities you can draw between the experiences of these two individuals?

---

# CHAPTER 9

# Living with MS and stroke: a carer's perspective

*Gill Ayling*

*This chapter explores the challenges faced by those who care for someone with a long-term condition. What follows is a personal, sensitive and sometimes emotional account of the realities of being a carer; exploring what it means to be a carer and the impact it has on quality of life. The chapter deals with a variety of themes, including the impact of diagnosis, relationships, coping strategies, and personal expectations and aspirations, and also looking at ongoing healthcare provision and relationships with health and social care services. Gill is the main carer for her husband Mike. Mike is 62 years old and was diagnosed with multiple sclerosis (MS) at the age of 45 years. He also suffered a stroke at 58 years of age.*

> Multiple sclerosis is a condition of the central nervous system characterized by damage to the myelin sheath surrounding the nerve fibres. Nerve impulses travelling to and from the brain and spinal cord are consequently distorted or interrupted.
>
> Stroke is a brain injury caused by sudden interruption of blood flow to the brain. This may be ischaemic—the blood supply is stopped due to a blood clot—or haemorrhagic—a weakened blood vessel bursts.

The majority of people struggle to understand what it is truly like to be a carer. I hope these recollections and reflections of my personal experiences over the past 17 years will give you, the reader, a taste of 'our real life', and enable you to gain some insight into what it is really like to be the full-time carer for someone suffering from a long-term condition.

## Diagnosis

Looking back, we first noticed something was wrong when Mike couldn't walk properly, but it was so intermittent that he thought he had a trapped nerve. At this point, I think I was more worried than he was; I had looked up his symptoms in medical books and had got a vague idea that it could possibly be MS. Mike was referred to a consultant neurologist and sent for a magnetic resonance imaging (MRI) scan and other tests. At the time I tried to prepare him for the worst, but he refused to discuss it, convinced it was a trapped nerve. We went together for the results of the scan and the consultant was very blunt and matter-of-fact: 'You have got MS, the type we call primary progressive MS, and there is nothing we can do for you.' We tried to ask sensible questions and asked about the MS Society, but the consultant suggested that if we wrote to them they would send some information booklets, qualifying this by saying, 'I wouldn't bother going to the meetings, what you will find out will scare you to death. At this stage, just go away and get on with your life.' We left the hospital utterly shocked and not quite knowing what to do, and with no real support, just the promise of a follow-up appointment in a years' time.

I went home and prepared for the worst. I had read about Jacqueline Dupree, the famous cellist, being dead a year after diagnosis and I thought Mike was going to be in a wheelchair in a few months time. The MS Society sent out some booklets, including one to give to our son, who was only eight years old at the time. Mike was in denial and refused to read them and although I read them all, they just frightened me even more. Looking back, this was an awful time. We were left devastated with the feeling that there was absolutely no-one to talk to. I can remember ringing friends and family who were all very sympathetic, but then getting that feeling that they didn't believe me or that I had over-exaggerated when we met up, because when they saw him they saw a man with nothing visibly wrong. I think his mum found it the hardest to accept—she never did acknowledge that there was anything wrong with him. Even when his symptoms became more noticeable she would insist he drive the 20 miles to see her once a week. She would expect him to mow the lawn when he visited as he had always done, even though he could only mow our own lawn in stages otherwise his legs would give way. In those early years, I used to get the same feeling of disbelief in his disability from people we met when we went out. He would be in his wheelchair, talking, laughing and joking, and I would see people looking at him and thinking that there isn't much wrong with him. There doesn't seem to be any middle ground in peoples' expectations; you are either disabled or you are not. Even now, although the family accept him as being ill and disabled, they seem to have moved directly from thinking there is absolutely nothing wrong to his being 'past it'. When they come and see us, they don't talk to him but pat him on the head as if he isn't there.

At first, the changes were not very noticeable as the symptoms of the disease just affected his walking and the function of his bowels and bladder. His mobility problems were, in the beginning, quite manageable. Initially he just had to walk fast to keep his balance, which meant I used to follow in his wake as he went through town at full-speed, knocking into everyone and profusely apologizing, although gradually he came to need the wheelchair more and more. He would not, however, face up to the problems he had with the function of his bowel and bladder, and this was more challenging to cope with. If we met someone we knew when we were out, he would never break away from a conversation, admit he needed the toilet and excuse himself, but would wait until they left and often this was too late. Then we would be in an awful mess because we were in a public place; I would have to completely change and tidy him up after searching for the only disabled toilet I could find. There were occasions when I left him alone in a public toilet while hastily shopping for a complete set of clothes, towel and flannel. I always accepted his refusal to acknowledge this issue as a problem though, because I realized this was his way of coping with what he felt was the most distressing of his symptoms.

We coped quite well until he had to stop driving and finish work on the grounds of ill health. He was a car design engineer and his life revolved around cars. He loved cars—everything was very car-orientated, even outside of work he used to marshal for the grand prix in his spare time. He used to drive to work and take our son to school and college on the way, but finally even he refused to go with his dad because the driving was so dangerous. This came to a head when he had an accident and hit another car, although even then he would not listen to anyone or accept that he was not safe to drive. Eventually, I told the neurologist he was not fit to drive. I felt terrible betraying him in this way, but I knew that I had no choice. Before he lost his driving licence there had been concerns at work. He had one or two embarrassing accidents having lost control over his bladder and bowels, and his personality had started to change (his MRI scans at the time showed he had developed some brain lesions) and he started upsetting people at work without even realizing it. As a result, he had been asked on several occasions to consider taking early retirement. The combination of work-related issues and being unable to drive culminated in a long period of sick leave and he subsequently took retirement for ill health, even though he was still only 54 years old, but this loss of independence magnified the problems he was having. It was as though someone had told him 'you're now disabled', and in his mind he completely agreed and began to act that way. He lost his motivation, would no longer do anything to help himself and for me, it felt as if things started to go rapidly downhill. Eventually we took the decision to move from a house to a bungalow to make things easier and he started to attend a day centre to give me a break.

## Relationships

MS changed our relationships; with each other as husband and wife, socially with friends, and as a family unit. Mike's personality gradually changed and he has now become someone I don't really know. As the years passed, I would always tell people the reason we were still together was because we had always had a good marriage, we had never experienced 'a rough period', and we just coped with the things life threw at us. We all know that a 'good marriage/relationship' is peppered with the irritating and 'niggling' personality traits that we dislike about our partner, but we put up with it because we love them and essentially they are minor issues in our lives. As the illness progressed, it was as if all these elements of Mike's personality came to the forefront and the nice bits that I loved him for seemed to disappear. Everything that I used to put up with as a minor irritation became a major irritation because these now dominated his personality.

Mike didn't change overnight; in fact, the changes in his personality were gradual. He was never really a very outgoing person and he always preferred to talk to people 'one-to-one' rather than in a crowd, but over time this changed to the point where he has stopped talking to people altogether, even if they speak to him first. He would upset friends because of the way he acted and the things he said, but had no idea of the effect he was having. I remember taking him out one day and he took me completely by surprise—the sun was shining and we had had a meal sitting outside a local pub. I thought to myself life isn't so bad, we can cope with this. He turned round, looked straight at me, and said, 'If I hadn't been ill I would have divorced you by now'. I thought to myself, 'he doesn't really mean that, he's just frustrated'. Later that day I told him that I was still feeling quite upset by what he had said, but it was if it had never happened and he couldn't even remember saying it.

Mike's relationship with our son was also changed by the illness. Jonathon looks back now and says he sometimes feels that he has not had a father because, unlike me he cannot remember the 'normal', good person that I married. Mike used to fall quite often, and when Jonathon was still living at home we would try and pick him up. He would swear frequently, curse and lash out at us, and often we would end up walking away and leaving him on the floor in a heap to calm down. Before the illness he was a man who never swore or cursed. I know that it was frustrating for both of us, trying not to retaliate and keep calm, and there were occasions when we would both lose our tempers with him.

Normal relationships do not always run smoothly, but you can retaliate and have an argument. This is not true for us. I remember on one occasion pushing him around town as he was being absolutely awful, rude, temperamental and argumentative, and I snapped back at him. People were glaring at me and I could see them thinking, 'who is this awful woman shouting at this poor man in a wheelchair?' It's then that you realize you can't shout at a disabled person in public. Then there is the other side of the coin, the constant frustration at your own situation. Sometimes I lose control over my emotions and become someone I don't recognize. I remember being so cross and frustrated on one occasion that I slapped him—it was so out of character for me, I felt so guilty and ashamed that I went to the doctor and confessed. There is not really a husband–wife relationship between us now—that closeness has gone. I don't think he even kisses me anymore. Essentially, the relationship has become very one-sided and selfish; he sees me as the carer, someone who is only there to look after him.

## Personal expectations and aspirations

I feel a sense of loss and regret for what might have been when I look at our life as it is now. How do you see yourself in years to come as you approach retirement? How did I see myself as a woman in her 60s? When I married Mike, he was the sort of person I could imagine still having a good conversation with as we grew older together; I always thought that we would have plenty to talk about. We used to share everything, but that has vanished because I am married to someone who I no longer really know and who doesn't really respond to me. I envisaged that we would travel a lot as we got older and have more freedom from work. We both loved to travel and loved our holidays; even when Mike started using a wheelchair we still planned to go away each weekend and go to places in the country. As everyone does, we mapped out a plan of the life we were going to lead (our son was, by this time, at university); we thought we would get out and about, and go here, there and everywhere.

Now I feel trapped and frustrated. I know it isn't Mike's fault and I look around and see people much worse off than myself. But as a carer, your life stops and I can't really see a future. I often find myself wondering what the point is, that there is no future; I feel that I have become an old woman before my time. Deep down I want to be able to go out, go on holiday, see and experience different things and feel as if *I* am 'normal' again. It worries me thinking about what might be and I become stressed and anxious if I spend too long thinking about the future; it is so much easier to concentrate on the here and now. I realize that I might not always be able to care for Mike at home, and that arranging for him to go into a nursing home is one of the options, but this is a big decision and I don't feel this is the right choice for us just yet.

## Health and social care services

Living with and caring for someone with a long-term condition inevitably means contact with a wide range of health and social care professionals and services; all of which you are led to believe are in place for the patient's and carer's benefit and ultimately, to improve your quality of life. Although on the whole this is true and Mike and I have always been grateful for the help we have been given and receive—negotiating a path through this complex process has never been easy.

Accessing the help and services you need at the time you need it always seems to be difficult. In the early days, after Mike finished work we didn't need much help because we could manage to do the everyday things like assisting him to stand. As a family we coped on our own, occasionally getting the neighbours in if he had a 'bad' day. Eventually though, Mike had more and more 'bad' days; he was increasingly falling and we felt we were asking too much of our neighbours. It was then that we found out that it wasn't that there was no help available to us, we just didn't seem to be able to access it. A variety of professionals (e.g. social worker, physiotherapist, occupational therapist) would come out to assess Mike's physical capabilities to see whether he could stand or walk without wobbling. They would make their notes, nod agreeably and leave, but within minutes Mike would be wobbling unsteadily around the living room and down he would go on the floor again. It got so bad that eventually we were ringing an ambulance up to five times a week. I always felt guilty for calling them out, it felt like everyone seemed to be cross with us. It happened so frequently that we got to know the paramedics personally. Most of them were nice, apart from one crew who we dreaded because they would always criticize us, saying we shouldn't be calling them and what we needed was to get some more help, when all the time we were desperately trying to do just that. I remember one incident when Mike ended up with carpet burns on his bottom, because I had felt so guilty about calling the ambulance that I made him shuffle across the floor to get to his chair.

This 'merry-go-round' of never quite getting the help we really needed seemed to last forever. Therapists would keep coming out to reassess him and each time they would suggest a new piece of equipment—'a banana board', 'a raise cushion'—but not the real and personal physical help we actually needed. They would spend time demonstrating each new piece of equipment and showing us how safe it could be. I can remember one young therapist who was very slightly built sitting on the top of an inflating cushion to demonstrate its stability, the reality with a slightly overweight MS sufferer was not quite as reassuringly secure.

Eventually the person who helped us to sort things out the most was our district nurse, who organized a meeting at the hospital with all of the different people involved with in Mike's care (GP, community matron, nurses, social workers, therapists, paramedics). It finally felt like Mike and I were given the opportunity to say what we wanted to happen with everyone there. They sorted out a proper package of care, regular help from home carers, and things like a ceiling track hoist. Even now, however, it is still not always plain-sailing. We have the help, services and equipment we need, but if anything changes things still seem to take too long to happen. People will agree we need a new piece of equipment, say they are going to get it, then they go away and you wait. In addition, there is the cost element— social services always seem to mention the cost of equipment and services and this can make you feel quite guilty. For example, it became increasingly difficult to sit Mike up in bed. The nurse and social worker agreed that it was perhaps time to get an electric hospital bed, but nothing happened. Tired of waiting, I bought a wedge and special cushions to help sit him up in bed. Mike has since developed a bed sore and the nurse told me this was because we started to use the wedge and cushions to sit him up in bed.

Good communication, or should I say a lack of, seems to be the greatest difficulty we have with health professionals. One of the biggest problems is that people do not seem to truly listen to what you say when they talk to you. One of the most frustrating things is that many health professionals make assumptions about Mikes' level of disability. They do not treat us as individuals with a greater level of knowledge and insight about what he can and cannot do. I remember one occasion taking Mike to outpatients to see the urologist, who asked me whether he could stand. I said 'no.' But he ignored me and said 'well we'll just get him on the couch.' Perhaps you can visualize the scenario; we ended up with Mike trying desperately to stand, the consultant on one side and nurse on the other, with me lifting his feet—the three of us hauling him like a sack of potatoes onto the couch. (Mike is no lightweight at 15 stone.) That was in a hospital environment where they must have equipment or a hoist, but they can't seem to be bothered to get them.

Communicating with agencies to obtain financial support and allowances has also been difficult. Obtaining disability living allowance (DLA) was a problem, as we kept being refused initially. The endless paperwork and forms did not reflect what Mike could and could not do, and the assessor we had never properly examined Mike. As a result we were awarded just a fraction of the full allowance. We were told we could challenge the decision, but this meant going to a tribunal. I did ring to ask what this would involve but was told, 'you can pursue this but we know the sort of people who are swinging the lead, we can suss them out and you are unlikely to get the decision changed.' This made us feel terrible, as if we were trying to obtain money under false pretences, but Mike was genuinely disabled. The GP was really good at this time and helped us out. He spoke to the benefits office and asked for copies of the assessor's report in which it transpired that he/she had stated: 'The wife states he has primary progressive MS, a term I have not of heard before. He shows no physical signs of being disabled.' The GP sent further reports and explained Mike's level of disability and diagnosis. As a result, the benefits office apologized saying that the report had given no indication of the problems we were having and that we would now be allocated both carer's and mobility allowances.

## Coping strategies

Now Mike is more dependant, I get help every day from social services and have regular home carers coming twice every day, seven days a week. Mike goes to a day centre three days a week. He leaves around 10 am and returns at around 3.30 pm. As a consequence, our days are very regimented and organized with military precision. The days on which Mike goes to day care are supposed to be 'me time', to give me a bit of a break, but often all I can do is use them to catch up with shopping and housework. They are very limiting as everything I choose to do on these days has to be organized to fit around the restricted five-hour time-slot. I have tried a variety of activities on these days; I joined a gym recently, but fitting it in is a bit of a struggle and it can be lonely going on your own, I tried the University of the Third Age, but any courses and activities they have always seem to fall outside of my available time. Sometimes I go to a garden centre with my neighbour, but we can't travel too far because I have to get back for Mike and you are always aware of the time. My social worker said they wanted to meet my needs as well as Mike's. She said: 'We want to give you time, whatever you would like to do, we can make it happen, whatever you would find relaxing.' I told them that what I'm really interested in is bird watching and that I would love to go on a day trip with the Royal Society for the Protection of Birds (RSBP), and they said that they could arrange that. I got quite excited and obtained all the details. The trips left around 8 am and got back at around 6 pm—it was then that they told me the timing was too long.

One good thing about social services is that I do get some respite care—I am allowed up to four weeks respite in a year, but it was struggle to get this at first. It was at a period when I felt I had hit 'rock bottom'; social services had come out to the house for a meeting with the care workers who were saying that I needed more help and social services were arguing that I didn't. My son was there too, as he had taken the day off work. Halfway through the meeting I thought that no-one was actually listening to me. I stood up and told them so. I was going to make a grand gesture of getting into my car and driving off into the sunset. I nearly did it too, but when I actually got outside the social worker had blocked me in with his car. Instead, I sneaked across to my neighbour's home and waited until all the cars had gone. They decided I needed regular respite care after this, but it shouldn't be like this. I didn't want to be one of those people who threw a tantrum to get what they want, but I felt driven to it.

Although the respite care gives me a much-needed break it is only four weeks out of 52 and organizing it can be quite stressful. There are so many rules and regulations. Social workers tell me that respite care is supposed to be used when I really need it (i.e. when I am close to breakdown), but I don't see it like that; it is too late then and I don't get any benefit from the break. That first time when I walked out of the meeting, they put Mike in a nursing home for a week to give me a break, but all I did was sit at home crying for most of the time. I need respite to get away from it all and to be able to mix with ordinary people. If I can, I like to use some of my respite entitlement to book a holiday and get away abroad, but this is always difficult as the regulations will not let me arrange the time too far in advance, which means I get caught in the trap of leaving my booking till the last minute and then not being able to book anything at all. I did manage to take a 'real' holiday last year; I went to Slovenia with my son and we did a lot of walking, something I always used to enjoy. It felt so good, to do things I hadn't done for years. Inevitably, once you return, reality comes crashing down. I know that my son will not always want to take me away and I know I still can't do anything on the spur of the moment, or even on a regular or weekly basis, unless it fits around day care and its limited schedule.

There are support groups to help you cope and these can be helpful for some people. It can give you an opportunity to talk to other people who understand what it is like to be a carer, but there is a part of me that doesn't want to join such groups. I want to be a normal person and meet normal people with normal families. Being a carer can be very lonely and isolated; I sometimes feel I don't have anyone to talk to now that my son has left home. You learn to keep a lot of your worries to yourself. People are always sympathetic and ask you how you are and I would respond by pouring it all out to them, but they don't really want to know. You can very quickly lose your friends if you always ring them to moan. We have lost a lot of friends over time, but the good ones have stayed the course.

I began by saying that most people don't truly know what it is like to be a carer; they can't imagine what it is like nor understand what you are going through. Everyone judges as they see. They look no further than the image they get from a man in a wheelchair; they do not see the person pushing the chair. On a bad day, if you asked me if there was one word I would use to describe being a carer, it would be 'despair'. Despair that in spite of the services and people we get help from, overall you are on your own all the time. I think the words of my son as a young boy (only a couple of years after Mike's diagnosis) sum up the true impact of living with a long-term condition, when he said, 'It isn't just dad that's got MS is it mum? It's all of us'.

*Gill's experiences highlight the challenges and problems that frequently face those who become long-term carers of family members. The impact of being a carer and the changes this has meant have influenced every aspect of Gill's daily life. It is also clear that this is has not only affected Gill, but her family as well, and on a variety of levels: physically, socially, psychologically, and environmentally. It has impacted on all her relationships: personal, familial, social, and with health and social care professionals. She has clearly highlighted the difficulties that carers face when negotiating with a myriad of services and agencies, and how this can impact on the quality of care for both patient and carer.*

*Her account raises some interesting points for consideration from a nursing perspective: the importance of effective communication between professionals and carers, and also inter-professionally between the agencies involved; the importance of ensuring that, where possible, appropriate services, adaptions and equipment are coordinated to provide the seamless delivery of care, which focuses on improving the quality of life for both patient and carer; and the relevance of thinking ahead where long-term care is anticipated, in order to effectively plan and prioritize for ongoing care and services.*

*As a nurse, it is important to develop the ability to look holistically at the needs of the carer, as well as the patient, and to acknowledge their personal values, aspirations and expectations.*

---

**Reflection**

- Think about carers you have met
- Have you always considered their needs along with those of the patient?
- Try developing a 'listening' approach that respects the contribution and knowledge that the carer or patient has as the 'expert' in his/her own circumstances
- Do you always involve them in negotiating and planning for the care provided?
- You might like to read this chapter in conjunction with the previous chapter which explores the experiences of a patient
- Are there any similarities in the aspects care and quality of life issues that were most challenging to both Gill and Tony?

---

# Further information

*MS Society: www.mssociety.org.uk*

*The Third Age Trust is the national representative body for the Universities of Third Age (U3As) in the UK. U3As are self-help, self-managed lifelong learning cooperatives for older people no longer in full-time work, providing opportunities for their members to share learning experiences in a wide range of interest groups and to pursue learning not for qualifications, but for fun: www.u3a.org.uk*

# CHAPTER 10

# Dementia

*Chris Knifton*

When considering the term 'dementia', it is important to note that this is in fact an umbrella term, used to describe a set of symptoms, which include a variety of causes (e.g. Alzheimer's disease—the most common form of dementia). The number of people diagnosed in the UK with dementia is estimated at 683 597, and current figures suggest by the year 2021, 940 110 people will have been diagnosed (Knapp and Prince, 2007). Dementia costs the UK £17 billion each year (Department of Health [DH], 2009a). The majority of care provision for people with dementia is provided through primary care services (Petit, 2005), with two thirds of all people with dementia living in their own homes (DH, 2009a). Although the majority of people with dementia are older people, there are at least 15 000 people under the age of 65 years with dementia (Knapp and Prince, 2007). There is, at present, no cure for dementia, and in Alzheimer's disease the average life expectancy from symptom onset can range from two to over 16 years (Corey-Bloom and Fleisher, 2005).

Despite dementia being a long-term condition, unfortunately there remains a low-level of non-specialist understanding, with a generally low priority attached to the development of appropriate care skills (All-Party Parliamentary Group on Dementia, 2009; DH, 2009a). The aim of this chapter is to provide an understanding of some of the issues that may affect the lives and experiences of people with dementia following diagnosis, and the role of non-specialist nurses who come into contact with this patient group. By reading this chapter, and through personal reflection, the following learning outcomes can be achieved:

* A basic understanding of the term dementia and its common symptoms
* Understanding the role of different professionals supporting the person with dementia and his/her family
* Insight into applying biopsychosocial frameworks to understand how long-term conditions, such as dementia, may be individually experienced
* Reflection on how individual practice can positively support and 'make a difference' to a person's experience of dementia.

A number of reports have echoed the concerns felt by many that the care for people with dementia continues to remain unsatisfactory (*Table 10.1*). These reports show that dementia is gathering increasing social concern in the UK. However, they also recognize that dementia should not be seen as an inevitable part of ageing, and that if it does occur, much can still be done to help people, whatever stage of the condition they may be at (National Institute for Health and Clinical Excellence [NICE] and Social Care Institute for Excellence [SCIE], 2006; DH, 2009a).

# What is dementia?

Dementia is often described as an 'umbrella term'. It is defined as:

> *'A syndrome due to disease of the brain, usually of a chronic or progressive nature, in which there is disturbance of multiple higher cortical functions, including memory, thinking, orientation, comprehension, calculation, learning capacity, language and judgement. Consciousness is not clouded. Impairments of cognitive functioning are commonly accompanied, and occasionally preceded by deterioration in emotional control, social behaviour or motivation.'*
>
> World Health Organization (1992: 49)

---

### Table 10.1 Published reports on the care of people with dementia

---

- *Forget me not* (Audit Commission, 2000)
- *National Service Framework for Older People* (Department of Health, 2001a)
- *Everybody's Business* (Care Services Improvement Partnership, 2005)
- *Dementia: Supporting people with dementia and their carers in health and social care* (National Institute for Health and Clinical Excellence and Social Care Institute for Excellence, 2006)
- *Dementia UK* (Knapp and Prince 2007)
- *Improving Services and Support for People with Dementia* (National Audit Office, 2007)
- *Living Well with Dementia: National Dementia Strategy for England* (Department of Health, 2009a)
- *Prepared to Care: Challenging the dementia skills gap* (All-Party Parliamentary Group on Dementia, 2009)

---

**Table 10.2 Common symptoms of dementia**

---

- Memory loss, particularly with short-term memory
- Orientation problems
- Aphasia (partial or total loss of the ability to articulate ideas or comprehend spoken or written language) and other communication difficulties
- Apraxia (total or partial loss of the ability to perform coordinated movements or manipulate objects)
- Agnosia (loss of the ability to interpret sensory stimuli, such as sounds or images)

Although less common, additional symptoms may also include:
- Changes in personality
- Complex or difficult behaviours, sometimes referred to as behavioural and psychological symptoms, which may include aggression; delusions; depression; hallucinations; mental ill-health; psychosis; sexual disinhibition; shouting/excessive vocalization; what may appear as inappropriate walking/restlessness

---

Dementia, Burns et al (2002: 10) write, is not a diagnosis, but a 'clinical description of a cluster of signs and symptoms'. A variety of attempts have been made to group together these signs and symptoms, including the use of categories such as neuropsychological, neuropsychiatric, and problems in carrying out the activities of daily living (Burns et al, 2002). Overall, however, the term dementia is used to describe a group of symptoms that result from the destruction of brain cells (Brotchie, 2003). Some common general symptoms are shown in *Table 10.2*, although these symptoms will vary according to the individual, the form of dementia, and stage of the disease.

---

**Reflection**

- Consider what the term 'dementia' signifies to you
- How would you feel as a student nurse being asked to care for a person with a diagnosis of dementia?
- Do you feel comfortable, relieved, anxious, frightened, well-prepared, challenged?
- Your feelings may be based on preconceptions, presumed competence, or past/current experiences; this affects how we feel we may be able to react to, and provide assistance with, the varying symptoms of dementia.

---

All forms of dementia are progressive, and some people think of this progression as a series of early, middle and late (or advanced) stages. In the early stage, short-term memory loss, poor judgement, and loss of interest are clear features. The middle stages are characterized by increasing memory and language problems, and a greater need for assistance with everyday activities, and sometimes behavioural and psychological symptoms, such as agitation or hallucinations. In the late or advanced stages, the person will become increasingly frail with mobility problems and communication difficulties clearly evident. Behavioural and psychological symptoms may worsen, or sometimes may even appear to diminish. Increasing support with the activities of daily living will be required, as well as assistance with any physical health problems that may include dysphagia (difficulty swallowing), weight loss, incontinence, infections and tissue viability.

However, there remains a danger of viewing the course of dementia as a natural progression through a series of stages. Some stages may overlap, with the inevitable consequence of symptoms appearing at stages other than would be usually expected. Marshall and Tibbs (2006) note that people with dementia will experience these stages to different degrees, with some stages sometimes not experienced at all.

There are many different forms of dementia (*Table 10.3*), although many share these common symptoms, particularly as the condition progresses.

### Alzheimer's disease

Alzheimer's disease is the most common cause of dementia in the Western world (McCabe, 2008). The number of people with the condition is slightly higher in women than men (Jorm, 2005), with prevalence increasing with age. In a very small number of cases, a familial or genetic link can be found. For people with Down's syndrome, a common form of learning disability,

---

**Table 10.3 Common forms of dementia and incidence**

- Alzheimer's disease (60% of cases)
- Vascular dementia (20% of cases)
- Mixed (Alzheimer's and vascular dementia)
- Dementia with Lewy bodies (15%)
- Other (e.g. alcohol-related dementia, Creutzfeldt-Jakob disease, frontotemporal lobe dementia)

From: Department of Health (2001a)

---

there is also an increased risk of Alzheimer's (Kerr, 2007). Alzheimer's disease usually has a slow onset with a gradual progression (Corey-Bloom and Fleisher, 2005; Adams, 2008). Memory loss, particularly for recent events, is a key concern. A common feature is the need for relatives/carers to repeat answers to asked questions, or the frequent misplacement of everyday objects. Problems that gradually emerge include judgement, orientation and language difficulties. Relatives or neighbours may also show concern over forgetful behaviour leading to risk, such as leaving the gas cooker unlit but turned on, or food left on the cooker until it burns. Global deterioration steadily develops, resulting in problems with continence, mobility, eating/drinking, and swallowing. Together, the variety of symptoms affects the ability to carry out daily activities, with a loss of independence, leading to additional problems for the individual and his/her family. Missed appointments, getting lost on familiar routes, misplaced and/or inappropriately stored items in the home, may all become increasingly apparent. Behavioural disturbances can occur early, but tend to become more frequent as the severity of dementia increases (NICE/SCIE, 2006). Such symptoms may include agitation, hallucinations, delusions or aggression. Increased physical dependence is apparent as the condition advances further.

---

### Case study I

*Over the past few months, Ms Timms has started to appear forgetful. She has missed planned social events with her friends, forgotten when her daughter is visiting, and missed a routine GP appointment. Her speech is quite repetitive at times, and her house is untowardly untidy. She often misplaces items, and sometimes finds them in quite unlikely places. Ms Timms has got lost in town twice while shopping, despite the route being a familiar 10-minute walk. Her daughter often complains that she has to repeat conversations to her mother and at times requires prompting for the simplest of routine activities.*

---

## Vascular dementia

Nielsen-Brown and Chui (2009) argue that vascular dementia is the second most common form of dementia, either on its own or coupled with Alzheimer's disease (mixed dementia). Incidence rates are initially higher in males then females (NICE/SCIE, 2006) and in certain ethnic groups, such as Japanese and Caribbean (Brown and Hillam, 2004). Generally, it is caused by a deficiency in oxygen to certain parts of the brain, usually following a stroke (cerebrovascular accident) or small vessel disease, with resulting symptoms of dementia. When, in the rare circumstances that dementia arises from a single stroke, it is referred to as 'single-infarct dementia'. However, it more commonly arises as a result of number of smaller strokes, where it may be referred to as 'multi-infarct dementia'. There are a number of different types of vascular dementia. Its course is often abrupt, and follows a step-wise progression. The patient may experience a sudden decline (following a stroke/series of mini-strokes), before a relative stable period (i.e. days, weeks or even months) until the next stroke. This makes the course of vascular dementia difficult to predict.

---

### Case study 2

*Mr Shilkoo developed hypertension (high blood pressure) when he was in his early 50s. He worked long hours as a book-keeper for a car manufacturer, and often appeared stressed. He smoked, was overweight, and took little exercise. In his mid-60s he had his first stroke and was admitted to the local hospital. He appeared to make a good recovery, although he was left with mild weakness to his left arm and some minor memory problems. One year later, Mr Shilkoo had a second stroke, this time being admitted to hospital for a longer period. On discharge, Mr Shilkoo's speech had become affected and memory problems became more pronounced. He also experienced increasing disorientation to both time and place. Following a third stroke six months later, Mr Shilkoo's memory difficulties significantly worsened, with both short- and long-term memory problems, where he required increased levels of support with his activities of daily living.*

---

## Dementia with Lewy bodies

McKeith (2005: 607) notes that by the 1990s, dementia with Lewy bodies was a 'relatively common cause of dementia in old age'. Autopsy studies indicate that this type of dementia currently accounts for 15–20% of dementias (Burn et al, 2009). Lewy bodies refers to the accumulation of abnormal proteins, occurring in the nerve cells of the brain. Dementia with Lewy bodies is associated with a progressive decline, although cognitive function can vary over minutes, hours, days, or even weeks. These can affect the ability to carry out the activities of daily living. Hallucinations are a common occurrence. Burn et al (2009) note that this may typically include visual hallucinations of adults, children or animals, as well as possible auditory hallucinations. Falls are often a regular feature, as is a shuffling gait. Dementia with Lewy bodies shares a number of clinical features with Parkinson's disease.

## Case study 3

*Mr Thomas, although physically well, had started getting headaches as well as experiencing memory problems. He experienced repeated falls at home and his walking became more 'shuffled'. On one occasion while sitting in the lounge, he clearly saw two children playing in the corner of the room. He called his partner, Jason, in alarm. Jason pointed out that there were no children there. Mr Thomas, however, was able to describe the children in very clear detail and also reported that he heard them laughing. In addition to this commonly repeated scenario, Jason reports that at times Mr Thomas can appear lethargic and generally disinterested, although will return to his 'usual self', sometimes a few hours or even a day later.*

## Other, often rarer forms of dementia

There are a number of rarer causes of dementia, including:

- Alcohol-related dementias and Korsakoff's syndrome
- Corticobasal degeneration
- Creutzfeldt-Jakob disease (CJD)
- Frontotemporal dementia (including Pick's diseases)
- HIV-associated dementia
- Huntington's disease.

The Alzheimer's Society produces a number of useful factsheets about the different forms of dementia, including some of the rarer types (http:// alzheimers.org.uk).

## Reflection

- Did you know there were many different forms of dementia?
- Although some of the more common symptoms present in all forms, some dementia types have very specific presentation with additional signs/symptoms
- Consider selecting one of the rarer forms of dementia that you may not have heard of or thought of as dementia
- Look at the fact sheet produced by the Alzheimer's society on this, or do some independent research in this area to widen your knowledge.

## Diagnosis

Before a diagnosis is made, other conditions that may present with similar symptoms of dementia should be ruled out. Although this list is not exhaustive, some of these may include:

- Brain tumours
- Constipation
- Dehydration
- Depression
- Effects/toxicity of drugs/substance misuse, alcohol or prescribed medication
- Infections
- Thyroid deficiencies
- Vitamin deficiencies
- Other delirium states.

Both recognition and understanding of depression and delirium in particular, with its range of causes, manifestations, and impact on long-term conditions, are essential to nurses working in this area. NICE are currently preparing guidelines for the recognition and management of delirium.

---

**Reflection**

- Consider what investigations can be undertaken to rule out treatable causes of dementia-like symptoms
- Think about the possible conditions listed. How are these diagnosed?
- Reflect on your knowledge of the causes of delirium and how this is investigated.

---

The process of reaching a diagnosis of dementia is not easy and a range of assessments of clinical presentation are required. These help not only in excluding potential treatable causes of the prevailing symptoms, but also identify additional problems both experienced and newly emerging. Diagnosis should be seen as a collaborative approach between the individual, carers/family members, and professionals actively involved in care provision, who together can provide information that may support a potential diagnosis. Such collaboration is paramount when one considers the time from first symptoms to diagnosis can be as much as 12 months (NICE/SCIE, 2006: 80).

Both the *National Service Framework [NSF] for Older People* (DH, 2001a) and NICE/SCIE (2006) suggest that following the appearance of symptoms, a detailed history of the person should be taken and include: presenting symptoms; medical/psychiatric history; substance misuse/alcohol history; behaviour/personality changes; and the accomplishment of activities of daily living. A thorough physical examination is required, which acts both to exclude other disorders, and also to document specific signs and symptoms. Blood tests that may help exclude delirium states are usually carried out. Medications, both prescribed and over-the-counter, are examined, including recent changes, side-effects, contraindications, withdrawal and possible toxicity. An examination of the person's overall mental state, including the presence or absence of psychiatric problems such as hallucinations, delusions, depression, and agitation, is required. Cognitive testing that includes establishing the true extent of cognitive impairment should be carried out using established rating scales such as the mini mental state examination (MMSE), abbreviated mental test score (AMTS), mental test score (MTS), Addenbrooke's cognitive examination (ACE), or clock-drawing test where appropriate. Such tests are designed to examine a range of memory, language, orientation, visuoperceptual, and object skills and recognition. Where necessary, structural imaging (computerized tomography [CT] and magnetic resonance imaging [MRI] brain scans), is considered. These may be used to detect the degree of atrophy or shrinkage in different areas of the brain, and may also be used to rule out possible brain tumours. In some cases, functional imaging (single photon emission computed tomography [SPECT] and positron emission tomography [PET] scans) may also be used, and are particularly useful if frontal lobe dementia is suspected.

The diagnosis of dementia is often made in primary care, generally with the type of dementia subsequently made by a specialist. Where a possible diagnosis of dementia is suspected, the person should always be referred to a memory assessment service/clinic as the single point of referral (NICE/ SCIE, 2006). Despite a notable diversity of such services provided under this title, what differentiates them from other services is their focus on the needs of people with dementia, and their families, particularly during the initial stage of the condition (Lindseay, 2008). This includes assessment, diagnosis, appropriate treatment, care, information and support (Luce et al, 2001).

Perhaps one of the early ethical dilemmas faced by health professionals during this process is who to tell if the diagnosis of dementia is confirmed. Marshall and Tibbs (2006) warn that when carers are told of the diagnosis, and the person with dementia is not, a greater strain on the relationship may occur, and the person with dementia can feel further isolated. Research indicates that the majority of people with mild dementia would wish to know their diagnosis, and best practice supports the view that clinicians 'discuss disclosure carefully with people with suspected dementia and their families to establish the best approach and what the person wishes to be told' (NICE/SCIE, 2006: 156).

## Understanding dementia: an enriched model

McCabe (2008) supports the view dementia is best understood, not solely as an organic condition, but rather as a condition with biomedical, psychological and social aspects. A 'helpful frame of reference' (Kitwood, 1993) to aid this way of understanding of dementia, also referred to as the 'enriched model of dementia' (Brooker, 2007), is illustrated through Kitwood's adoption of the equation:

$$D = P + B + H + NI + SP$$

*Kitwood (1993: 16)*

Kitwood argues that 'any individuals dementia (D) may be considered as the result of a complex interaction between five main components: personality (P), biography (B), physical health (H), neurological impairment (NI) and social psychology (SP)' (Kitwood, 1993):

- Personality. Brooker (2007: 50) notes that 'this refers to the totality of the strengths and vulnerabilities that we all carry with us as human beings, and that will have a direct effect on how an individual copes with the effects of their dementia'. Personality traits, temperament, phobias and anxieties are some examples
- Biography. This includes what has happened throughout the person's life: 'people make sense of what is happening to them in the here and now by reference to experiences they have had in the past' (Brooker, 2007: 49). Changes and losses, adventures and risks, opportunities and deprivations, and relationships, according to Kitwood (1993) are important elements
- Health. Although Kitwood (1993) originally called this physical health, it can also be expanded to include mental health. This is important when considering the number of people with dementia who also have depression or anxiety disorders (Ballard et al, 1996), as well as Kitwood's (1993) original concern with physical conditions that can cause confusion or complex behaviours that are a sign of pain or discomfort. NICE/SCIE (2006) report that people with dementia are at increased risk of physical health problems, and the consequences of such would no doubt affect the person's presentation
- Neurological impairment. This is closely related to the medical perspective and refers to problems with brain pathology, as a direct consequence of dementia. Through understanding the type or form of

dementia, and the effects that damage or atrophy to different parts of the brain might lead to, we are better able to understand the experience of dementia for the individual. Usually beginning with memory problems, as the dementia progresses more areas of the brain become affected, and the person's symptoms may increase. Neurological impairment to certain areas of the brain may explain behaviours such as sexual disinhibition and personality changes

- Social psychology. Brooker (2007) argues that this is the social and psychological environment in which people with dementia find themselves, which Kitwood (1993) describes as the person's individual experiences as he/she attempts to be, do, relate, and communicate, and the type of reaction received from others. Malignant social psychology (MSP)—the things that undermine personhood—is an important argument for why a person's experiences of dementia, and for some prevailing behavioural symptoms, vary. This includes disempowerment, mockery and infantilization. Brooker and Surr (2005) identify 17 different examples of MSP, but note that they are not usually carried out with malicious intent. However, the effect on the individual can often be substantial. The alternative to MSP is positive person work (Brooker and Surr, 2005), with some examples including empowerment, fun, and respect. As Brooker and Surr note (2005:18), 'with the onset of dementia individuals are very vulnerable to their psychological defences being attacked and broken down. As the sense of self breaks down, it becomes increasingly important that the sense of self is held within relationships that the person with dementia experiences ... the development of relationship occurs through the day-to-day interactions'.

This enriched model provides a suitable biopsychosocial framework to aid our understanding of dementia, and has been adopted in a variety of interventions and assessment tools, for example Dementia Care Mapping (Brooker and Surr, 2005) and the Pool Activity Level (PAL) Instrument (Pool, 2008).

---

### Reflection

- Take a moment to consider, despite the resources, work pressures or culture of care you find yourself working in, you can still have an impact on a person's quality of life through your day-to-day interactions
- Consider the effect of social psychology, both intentional and non-intentional on the people in your care, and the effect of this on their behavioural and psychological symptoms.

# Care management

The *NSF for Older People* (DH, 2001a) provides an example of a dementia care pathway. This begins with routine assessments and investigations to support diagnosis, usually followed or in conjunction with referral to a memory clinic and the community mental health team for older people. The local authority social services department will usually carry out a community care assessment, if one has not already been done. The legal basis for a community care assessment is found under the National Health Service and Community Care Act (DH, 1990). Its general purpose is to uncover the needs of the person and what services can be provided. For those aged 65 years and over, the single assessment process (SAP) is often used (DH, 2001a; 2002), with involvement from both health and social care agencies.

Carers are also entitled to an assessment. The largest proportion of care is usually provided by informal carers (spouses/partners, daughters/sons, relatives, friends/neighbours) who should be regarded as partners in dementia care (Brodaty et al, 2005). Marshall and Tibbs (2006) note that many carers are themselves older people, with Carers UK (2005) noting that 1.5 million carers are over the age of 60 years. The Carers (Recognition and Services) Act 2005 (DH, 1995) allows carers to request an assessment at the same time the person they are caring for is being assessed; The Carers and Disabled Children Act 2000 (DH, 2000) extends this right to assessment and services even if the person they are caring for declines the offer of an assessment; and The Carers (Equal Opportunities) Act 2004 (DH, 2004), also extends carers' assessments to include recognition of their choice to participate or continue in other activities such as work, education, or leisure. The Work and Families Act 2006 (Department of Trade and Industry [DTI], 2006) further extends support for carers in employment. Since 6 April 2007, carers have a legal right to 'request' flexible working when caring for an adult relative, such as changing hours or even working from home when practical. Finally, under the Employment Relations Act 1999 (DTI, 1999) carers have the right to take unpaid time off work for those they care for in cases of emergency. Continued support and detailed plans for enabling carers can be found in the Carers Strategy (DH, 2008).

Notably, Brotchie (2003) suggests that carers may have a variety of emotional reactions to the family member with dementia. These include feelings of protection, loss, shame, embarrassment, loneliness, isolation, anger, irritation, uncertainty, exhaustion and love, compassion and humour. As with many other long-term conditions, nurses have an important role in working alongside carers throughout the patient's journey, and providing them with additional support or directing them to the most appropriate professional or organization. *Table 10.4* provides a useful summary of the range of different

## Table 10.4 The multidisciplinary team

| Professional | Examples of role in dementia care |
|---|---|
| Alzheimer's Society | A charity for people with any form of dementia, not just Alzheimer's disease, and their carers. This can provide important information, help and support, and put people in touch with local support groups |
| Consultants (psychiatrist, neurologist) | Decisions about diagnosis (including evaluation of findings of investigations and diagnosis of dementia sub-type) and treatment, including medication regimens. Will usually have ultimate responsibility for care |
| Dietician | Nutritional assessment, advice on supplements and interventions for both weight loss and gain |
| GP | Often the first point of contact, and remains responsible for general health throughout the patient journey. Arrange initial assessments and investigations, often to rule out other causes, and make any necessary referrals. Some GPs may continue to monitor people placed in residential care on antipsychotic medication |
| Home carers | May be private or social services based. Provides assistance with essential tasks that may include washing, bathing, dressing, and/or medication prompts. There may be other tasks, depending on a needs assessment, for example essential cleaning or shopping. They are often commissioned by social services if need exists, and are based on local eligibility criteria. Direct payments, where the local authority instead gives money to the individual so services, including home care, can be individually purchased and provide individuals with greater choice and flexibility. However, certain conditions exist for this to be put in place, which the social worker will be able to advise on |
| Community psychiatric nurse/ community mental health nurse | Assessments of people at home and provide advice on coping strategies and interventions, mental health assessments, medication assessments, risk assessments, therapeutic |

| | |
|---|---|
| | interventions, health monitoring, education/ training, and care management |
| Admiral nurses | Admiral nurses are only available in some parts of the UK. Admiral nurses work solely with dementia patients and their carers, providing practical and psychological support, advice on interventions and coping strategies, as well as education on the condition |
| District/community nurses, specialist nurses | District nurses or community nurses may address the physical symptoms or complications of long-term conditions for those living at home. This may include continence assessments, management of physical conditions (such as diabetes), tissue viability concerns, palliative care and advice, health promotion, detection of possible delirium states |
| Other nurses | Nurses may also work within inpatient facilities (NHS assessment/treatment wards, nursing homes, nursing respite care facilities) or additional outpatient services (memory clinics, day hospitals) |
| Occupational therapist | Purposeful activities to maintain function in activities of daily living, environment adaptions, advice and support with cognitive skills |
| Other organizations | These include advocacy and support groups, befriending schemes, sitting services, day care, lunch clubs, laundry services, or chiropody, among others. The social worker or community nurse can advise on what is available locally |
| Physiotherapist | Promoting mobility for as long as possible, additional support as required, exercise, postural management (for eating/drinking, respiration, activities), moving and handling advice as needs change, assessment of gait |
| Psychologist | May be involved in the diagnosis, assistance in exploring complex (challenging) behaviours, and developing individualized therapeutic approaches/interventions |
| Respite placement providers | Sometimes also referred to as 'intermittent relief'. This may be in the form of day care, sitting services, or residential/nursing placement. Respite |

| | placements are designed to give the carer a break from caring, and also provide an opportunity for assessment where indicated |
|---|---|
| Social worker | Assessment of need and services, commissioning and access to certain services, risk assessment, case management, assistance with benefits, carers assessment, signposting to services/referrals |
| Speech and language therapist | Assessing and advising on swallowing difficulties, as well as effective communication strategies |

professionals who may be involved in this journey. The professionals listed, and their role, is not exhaustive, but provides a brief overview.

Presho (2008) suggests that case management is not about disease management in isolation, but rather about resolving complex issues in patients with multiple concerns. This is particularly important for progressive conditions with ever-changing needs and circumstances. The range of professionals and organizations reflect this complexity and the needs of the person with dementia and his/her carer(s).

## Reflection

- Consider your role in the care management of someone with a long-term condition such as dementia. Were you aware of the different professionals available and their role?
- As a nurse, consider your role working alongside someone from the multidisciplinary team. What knowledge might you have about an individual with dementia as a community nurse or student nurse that can be shared with the team to promote effective care management?

Following assessment, the NSF (DH, 2001a) pathway example for dementia outlines suggested treatment or care management options. Such services depend on the assessed health and social care needs of both the person with dementia and his/her carer. Examples of services available may include primary care services such as memory clinics, day hospitals and/or day centres, respite care/short breaks, carers support groups, counselling, or residential/nursing care, as well as hospital-based interventions and specialist treatment in both primary and secondary care services. NICE/

SCIE (2006) divides interventions commonly used in dementia care into the management of cognitive symptoms and non-cognitive (or 'behavioural and psychological') symptoms of dementia.

Cognitive symptoms are managed using both pharmacological and non-pharmacological approaches. NICE/SCIE (2006) provide a detailed account of the evidence in this area, describing non-pharmacological examples of communication strategies, memory books, skill training, assistive technology, reminiscence work, and reality orientation/cognitive stimulation as some examples. Pharmacological interventions include acetylcholinesterase inhibitors licensed to be used in mild to moderate Alzheimer's disease; memantine is also licensed for moderate to severe Alzheimer's (NICE/SCIE, 2006). Importantly, acetycholinesterase inhibitors and memantine are currently prescribed in forms of dementia other than Alzheimer's disease as part of a clinical trial only, or at clinical discretion without licence (NICE/SCIE, 2006: 186).

Non-cognitive symptoms of dementia may include agitation, aggression, shouting, sexual disinhibition, hallucinations, delusions, and 'wandering'. Approaches that may be considered may include aromatherapy, multi-sensory stimulation, therapeutic use of music/dancing, animal-assisted therapy, and massage (NICE/SCIE, 2006: 260–1). An individualized and tailored approach that takes into account the range of factors that might cause the behaviour is clearly advocated. This requires a comprehensive assessment that includes 'physical health, depression, pain/discomfort, medication side-effects, biography, psychosocial factors, environment and a behavioural/functional analysis' (NICE/SCIE, 2006: 260).

For non-cognitive symptoms, the use of pharmacological approaches are only advocated if the person with dementia is severely distressed or at immediate risk of harm, and when other strategies may prove ineffective. Any person on medication to manage behavioural and psychological symptoms requires careful monitoring and regular medication review. It is important that health professionals refer to the British National Formulary (BNF) (Joint Formulary Committee, 2009) and NICE/SCIE (2006) recommendations to guide their prescribing in this area. The side-effects of some medications may make the person's symptoms worse and/or lead to additional behavioural and psychological symptoms. McShane et al (1997) also found evidence supporting a poorer prognosis in people with dementia when antipsychotics were prescribed. In particular, care should be taken where a diagnosis of dementia with Lewy bodies is given.

It is perhaps fair to say that the majority of behavioural and psychological symptoms of dementia are in fact a form of communication. Through their actions, the person may be 'telling' us his/her story, that he/she is in pain, for example, feels lost and disorientated, or angry at our interventions. Marshall and Tibbs (2006) write that we are increasingly realizing that people with dementia are trying to communicate in whatever way they can. Different examples of specific communication difficulties that may lead to problems with normal communication may include:

- Dysphasia: receptive—difficulties in understanding what is being said; expressive—difficulties in producing words (Brocas aphasia); and nominal—finding the right word for a specific object
- Agnosia: difficulties in recognizing specific objects
- Prosopagnosia: inability to recognize familiar faces.

The presence of hallucinations and delusions and, as the dementia progresses, reduced control in using body language can have a profound effect. Some forms of dementia, such as frontotemporal dementia, may also have a specific 'communication' presentation, often involving language difficulties with dysphasia. Equally, there is a need to remember that the majority of people with dementia are older people. Sensory impairments (visual or auditory) common in this age group need careful consideration.

The Alzheimer's Society (2008) produces a useful factsheet on communicating with someone with dementia. This includes:

- Listen carefully to what the person has to say. If you are finding it difficult to understand the person, listen for clues and use what you know already about him/her to interpret carefully what he/she says
- Reduce, where possible, background noise and maintain eye contact in order to gain full attention
- Pay attention to the person's body language as he/she communicates. Consider the effect of your own body language and how this may be interpreted
- Speak clearly and calmly, using short sentences. Avoid asking direct questions, or asking the person to make complicated decisions. Allow time for the person to process information when you speak to him/her. Consider the impact of the tone of your voice
- Avoid contradiction. Consider how things appear to the person with dementia, their 'reality'
- Appropriate use of touch can be beneficial and provide needed reassurance
- Show respect at all times. Acknowledge the person as a person.

One must also consider how the person wishes to be addressed—first name, surname or otherwise. Reporting in both the nursing and national media (coverage November 2008 in response to planned NMC guidance

[2009]) has looked at the negatives of using inappropriate and often over-familiar terminology, such as 'dearie' and 'love'. Such 'terms of endearment' can be considered patronizing and unprofessional. For the person themselves, however, with or without dementia, this may be part of their usual speech architecture. This is evident through a regional use of differing terms across the country as greetings, displays of affection and perhaps more importantly, signs of community/group acceptance. Conflicts, however, exist over what is and what is not appropriate. The key is to address the person how he/she wants to be addressed, using terms he/she finds both socially and culturally appropriate, and that he/she feels are respectful.

Communication, respect and awareness of the effects of your actions/words can have a profound effect on the experiences we leave people with. This is true for any long-term condition, and dementia in particular.

---

### Reflection

• Consider the different ways your words/actions can make a positive difference to the people in your care
• Remind yourself each day when you start work: 'Today I can make a difference to their experience of the condition'.

---

## Self-management

Self-management, or self-care, is aimed at supporting individuals with long-term conditions to take control of their own health. It is an important element of the Expert Patient Programme (DH, 2001b), although there is debate as to how this can be appropriately applied to dementia care. Mountain (2006: 430) argues that equipping a person to cope with the challenges of 'medical management, maintenance, change and creation of meaningful roles, and the emotional consequences of a long-term condition', are central to self-management concepts. Requirements for self-management for people with dementia are (Mountain, 2006):

• Informing the person early on of his/her diagnosis
• Supporting the person with the consequences of diagnosis
• Focus on the needs of the person with dementia
• Identify specific interventions to facilitate self-management
• Professional education and support
• A whole-systems approach towards treatment and care.
  Mountain (2006: 441) notes that despite an emerging belief of

self-management in dementia, there is neglect of the possibilities and potential that this could provide, arguing 'the perquisites for self-management, namely disclosure of the diagnosis and a person-centred approach, are not always fulfilled by health and social care staff'. However, negative attitudes are changing and the possibilities that self-management may offer in dementia care are slowly becoming evident.

## Working with people with dementia in non-specialist adult settings

It is important that trained nurses do not feel outsiders to dementia care or lacking the appropriate skills, as warned by Adams (2008). There is, in fact, a clear role to be played by adult nurses in the care management of people with dementia. Detection of the early changes of dementia, for example, may occur when professionals become suspicious of unexplained changes in the individual. This may be apparent during routine visits when working in the community. The role of the nurse should include early recognition in patients of presenting symptoms that may indicate possible dementia, exclusion of other possible causes (for example delirium brought on by infections or uncontrolled disorders of metabolism), and prompt referral to the GP for further referral to a specialist service. Petit (2005) notes the importance of early recognition of symptoms so that a care plan, to include optimizing quality of life and appropriate treatment targeted at disease progression, can be delivered.

In addition, nurses working in primary care may be best placed to observe individuals who may be at greater risk of developing dementia. Petit (2005) notes the potential overlap in characteristics of patients at risk of coronary heart disease to that of dementia, arguing the potential for targeted interventions to prevent some dementias.

Indeed, when taken together, vascular dementia and mixed dementia types may account for up to 50% of all dementia cases (DH, 2009a). If physical health promotion strategies could reduce the numbers of people with certain types of dementia, then awareness among nurses of this important role should be encouraged. Adult nurses and students have long held an active role in health promotion, and are ideally placed to support cerebrovascular health initiatives. This includes advice on smoking cessation, diet and exercise. By explaining the risks not only of cerebrovascular problems, but also of vascular dementias, the impact of such campaigns would no doubt be increased (DH, 2009a). Research also exists to support the claim that vascular risk factors may be involved in Alzheimer's disease (Jorm, 2005), further increasing the potential of such campaigns. An additional list of 'modifiable factors' that may increase the risk of dementia, emphasizes the key role that adult nurses have in health promotion (NICE/SCIE, 2006):

- Alcohol consumption
- Smoking
- Obesity
- Hypertension
- Hypercholesterolaemia (raised cholesterol)
- Head injury
- Homocysteine levels, raised by low folate levels
- Exercise.

As argued by Adams (2008: 20), nursing people with dementia is indeed 'every nurse's business'. This is echoed in the *National Dementia Strategy for England* (DH, 2009a), which states that dementia must be seen as 'core business' for a number of services that the adult nurse may find him/herself in—including general practice and community nursing.

The role of nurses working in secondary care includes an awareness of challenges that the hospital environment may cause and to seek innovative ways of addressing this. Packer (2001) notes problems in relation to the design of the environment, the usual busy nature of a ward, and general poor understanding of dementia. Gathering comprehensive information from relatives about the person, including likes and dislikes, routine, important biographical details/life history, culture, and communication strategies can have a profound impact on the patient's experience of his/her hospital stay, and on the nursing staff. The DH (2009a) makes improving the quality of care in general hospitals a key objective in its National Strategy, to:

- Identify leadership for dementia in general hospitals
- Develop, in consultation with social services and key stakeholders, a care pathway for dementia
- Commissioning a specialist liaison older persons mental health team to work in general hospitals.

On discharge from general hospitals, some people may be transferred to a community hospital for rehabilitation or recuperation before final discharge home. This is sometimes referred to as intermediate care. Nurses working in these areas need to have the necessary skills and competencies about dementia just as much as those working in primary and secondary care. The DH (2009a) makes improving intermediate care for people with dementia another of its key objectives in its National Strategy, where:
- Care is accessible to people with dementia, and which meets their needs

- The needs of people with dementia need to be explicitly included and addressed in the revision of the DH guidance on intermediate care (2001c; 2009b).

## Conclusion

This chapter aims to present a brief introduction to dementia for student nurses and adult nurses with little previous knowledge about this condition. There remains a growing wealth of literature on this topic, and it has been difficult to synthesize the key aspects into just one chapter. Consideration, however, has been given to understanding the term dementia, routes to diagnosis, management of the condition, and the potential role of adult nurses working in this area, particularly nurses working in the community. Person-centred approaches that recognize the individual and uniqueness of their experience are central to care-management practices. Biopsychosocial frameworks, such as the enriched model of care, provide examples of doing this.

Working with people who have dementia may present many challenges, but also many opportunities. Both collectively as a nursing profession and as individuals, it remains within our power to make a lasting difference to a person's experience within our care. Our choice is what difference we now choose to make.

Adams T (2008) *Dementia Care Nursing: Promoting Well-being in people with Dementia and Their Families*. Palgrave Macmillan, Hampshire

All-Party Parliamentary Group on Dementia (2009) Prepared to care: Challenging the dementia skills gap. http://tinyurl.com/yzc8gkp (accessed 3 November 2009)

Alzheimer's Society (2008) Communicating. www.alzheimers.org.uk/factsheet/500 (accessed 3 November 2009)

Audit Commission (2000) Forget Me Not: Mental Health Services for Older People. http://tinyurl.com/ybmak22 (accessed 3 November 2009)

Ballard C, Bannister C, Solis M, Oyebode F, Wilcock G (1996) The prevalence, associations and symptoms of depression amongst dementia sufferers. *J Affect Disord* **36**(3–4): 135–44

Brodaty H, Green A, Low L (2005) Family carers for people with dementia. In: Burns A, O'Brien J, Ames D. eds, *Dementia*. 3rd edn. Hodder Arnold, London

Brooker D, Surr C (2005) *Dementia Care Mapping: principles and practice*. University of Bradford, UK

Brooker D (2007) *Person-centred dementia care: making services better*. Jessica Kingsley Publishers, London

Brotchie J (2003) *Caring for someone with dementia*. Age Concern England, London

Brown J, Hillam J (2004) *Dementia: your questions answered*. Churchill Livingstone, London

Burn D, Perry E, O'Brien J et al (2009) Dementia with Lewy Bodies. In: Charney DS, Nestler EJ. eds, *Neurobiology of mental illness*. 3rd edn. Oxford University Press, Oxford

Burns AS, Purandare N, Craig S (2002) *Mental Health in Older People in Practice*. Royal Society of Medicine Press Ltd, London

Carers UK (2005) Older Carers in the UK. http://tinyurl.com/ycgg8ql (accessed 3 November 2009)

Care Services Improvement Partnership (2005) Everybody's business. Integrated mental health services for older adults: a service development guide. http://tinyurl.com/ydzb9qm (accessed 3 November 2009)

Corey-Bloom J, Fleisher A (2005) The natural history of Alzheimer's disease. In: Burns A, O'Brien J, Ames D. eds, *Dementia*. 3rd edn. Hodder Arnold, London

DH (1990) *National Health Service and Community Care Act: Community care in the next decade and beyond*. DH, London

DH (1995) *The Carers (Recognition and Support services) Act*. DH, London

DH (2000) *Carers and Disabled Children Act*. DH, London. ref: 2000

DH (2001a) *National Service Framework for Older People*. DH, London. ref: 2001

DH (2001b) *The expert patient: a new approach to chronic disease management for the 21st century*. DH, London. ref: 2001

DH (2001c) *Intermediate care*. DH, London. ref: 2001

DH (2002) *Single assessment process: assessment tools and scales*. DH, London. ref: 2002

DH (2004) *Carers (Equal Opportunities) Act*. DH, London

DH (2008) *Carers at the heart of the 21st century families and communities: a caring system on your side, a life of your own*. DH, London

DH (2009a) *Living well with dementia: A National Dementia Strategy*. DH, London. ref: 11198

DH (2009b) *Intermediate Care: Halfway House*. DH, London

DTI (1999) *Employment Relations Act*. DTI, London

DTI (2006) *Work and Families Act*. DTI, London

Joint Forumulary Committee (2009) *British National Formulary* 58. September. BMJ Publishing Group Ltd and RPS Publishing, London

Jorm AF (2005) Risk factors for Alzheimer's disease. In: Burns A, O'Brien J, Ames D. eds, *Dementia*. 3rd edn. Hodder Arnold, London

Kerr D (2007) *Understanding learning disability and dementia: developing effective interventions*. Jessica Kingsley Publishers, London

Kitwood T (1993) Discover the person, not the disease. *J Dement Care* **1**(1): 16–17

Knapp M, Prince M (2007) *Dementia UK*. Alzheimer's Society, London

Lindseay J (2008) Memory clinics. In: Jacoby R, Oppenheimer C, Dening T, Thomas A. eds, *Oxford Textbook of Old Age Psychiatry*. Oxford University Press, Oxford

Luce A, McKeith I, Swann A, Daniel S, O'Brien J (2001) How do memory clinics compare with traditional old age psychiatry services? *Int J Geriatr Psychiatry* **16**(9): 837–45

Marshall M, Tibbs MA (2006) *Social work and people with dementia*. Policy Press, Bristol

McCabe L (2008) A holistic approach to caring for people with Alzheimer's disease. *Nurs Stand* **22**(42): 50–6

McKeith I (2005) Dementia with lewy bodies: a clinical overview. In: Burns A, O'Brien J, Ames D. eds, *Dementia*. 3rd edn. Hodder Arnold, London

McShane R, Keene J, Gedling K et al (1997) Do neuroleptic drugs hasten cognitive decline in dementia? Prospective study with necroscopy follow up. *BMJ* **314**(7076): 266–70

Mountain G (2006) Self-management for people with early dementia. *Dementia* **5**(3): 429–46

National Audit Office (2007) Improving services and support for people with dementia. http://tinyurl.com/dneog2 (accessed 3 November 2009)

NICE/SCIE (2006) Dementia: Supporting people with dementia and their carers in health in social care. http://guidance.nice.org.uk/CG42 (accessed 3 November 2009)

Nielsen-Brown N, Chui HC (2009) Vascular dementia. In: Charney D, Nestler E. eds, *Neurobiology of mental illness*. 3rd edn. Oxford University Press, Oxford

NMC (2009) *Guidance for the Care of Older People*. NMC, London

Packer T (2001) From the outside looking in: recognising skill in dementia care. *J Dement Care*. March/April: 29–30

Petit B (2005) The role of primary care in the management of dementia. In: Burns A, O'Brien J, Ames D. eds, *Dementia*. 3rd edn. Hodder Arnold, London

Pool J (2008) *The Pool Activity Level (PAL) Instrument for Occupational Profiling: A Practical Resource for Carers of People with Cognitive Impairment*. 3rd edn. Jessica Kingsley Publishers, London

Presho M (2008) Policy and Practice. In: Presho M. ed, *Managing Long Term Conditions: A Social Model for Community Practice*. Wiley-Blackwell, West Sussex

World Health Organization (1992) *The ICD-10 Classification of Mental and Behavioural Disorders. Clinical descriptions and diagnostic guidelines*. WHO, Geneva

# Useful websites

*www.ageconcern.org.uk*
*www.alzheimers.org.uk*
*www.carersuk.org.uk*
*www.cjdsupport.net*
*www.dlf.org.uk*
*www.hda.org.uk*
*www.helptheaged.org.uk*
*www.pdsg.org.uk*
*www.stroke.org.uk*

# CHAPTER 11

# Severe and enduring mental illness

*Jaqui Day, Paul Rigby and Teresa Pratt*

In a mental health context, long-term conditions are generally referred to as 'enduring or severe' mental health problems. The two main diagnoses which fall into this category are schizophrenia and bipolar affective disorder (previously known as manic depressive disorder). Although this chapter will begin with identifying the principal features which lead to a medical diagnosis, the main focus, by using a case study approach, will attempt to illustrate the biopsychosocial experience of living with an enduring mental health condition and the care that can be provided to meet the various, and often complex, needs of the individual.

Reading this chapter and reflecting on your own experiences should enable you to achieve the following learning outcomes:

• An understanding of the impact of schizophrenia and bipolar affective disorder on lifestyle and quality of life
• An understanding of the biopsychosocial model of care
• An understanding of the impact of stigma and discrimination
• To develop an awareness of the challenges faced by individuals with an enduring or severe mental health problem.

Schizophrenia and bipolar affective disorder are perhaps two of the most misunderstood and misinterpreted terms within the cannon of mental health conditions, but in a medical context the criteria for classification is fairly clear.

## Schizophrenia

According to the ICD-10, the classification manual most frequently used within European psychiatry, schizophrenia is generally characterized by 'distortions of thinking and perception and by inappropriate or blunted affect' (World Health Organization [WHO], 1992: 86). Schizophrenia is classed as a psychotic disorder and symptoms are divided into 'positive' and 'negative' which, in addition to causing distress, bewilderment and altered behaviour, generally impact on the characteristics that give us our feelings of 'individuality, uniqueness and self-direction' (WHO, 1992). Positive symptoms include experiences such as hallucinations (especially auditory), unusual beliefs (delusions), difficulty in thinking and concentrating, and sometimes feeling controlled (Royal College of Psychiatrists, 2004). Negative symptoms refer to a loss of interest, energy and emotions, and include 'apathy, paucity of speech and blunting or incongruity of emotional responses, usually resulting in social withdrawal and lowering of social performance' (WHO, 1992: 88). Schizophrenia usually begins between the ages of 15 and 35 years (slightly later in women) and will affect approximately one in 100 people (Royal College of Psychiatrists, 2004).

## Bipolar affective disorder

Although diagnostically, there are a number of different types of bipolar affective disorder, generally it is a condition characterized by severe mood swings. The mood can be low, manifesting as an intense depression with feelings of despair and hopelessness; or the mood can be high, manifesting as intense euphoria, over-activity, increased energy and loss of inhibition. Occasionally, these two extremes can coexist so the individual experiences a depressed mood with the increased energy, activity and restlessness associated with a manic state. Although bipolar affective disorder is classed as a mood disorder, sometimes when the mood swing is very severe psychotic features, such as hallucinations and delusions, might be evident. Manic episodes usually begin abruptly and last for between two weeks and five months. The average length of a depressive episode is six months (WHO, 1992). Bipolar affective disorder usually begins during or after the teenage years, and will affect approximately one in 100 people (Royal College of Psychiatrists, 2007).

## A model of care

While knowledge and awareness of the medical perspective is useful in terms of providing a shared language for understanding a cluster of signs and symptoms, it is only one aspect of these conditions as a whole. A model of care appropriate for individuals with serious mental health problems is the biopsychosocial model, which is a holistic view on health and sees the biological, psychological and sociological systems of the body as interconnected. Biological aspects of medication and medical treatment are not treated in isolation. Psychological and sociological factors, such as stress, culture, spirituality, beliefs, relationships, meaningful occupation, accommodation, and finances are treated as integral to the person and his/her recovery. The focus is on health and not on disease. This model was introduced by American psychiatrist George Engel (1977), and is reflected in the *National Service Framework for Mental Health* (Department of Health [DH], 1999), which requires an interdisciplinary approach to information gathering, while taking into consideration the patient's and carer's problems and needs, and identifying personal strengths and coping strategies.

---

### Case study I

*Kate is a 40-year-old female who lives in an affluent suburb. She has a long history of bipolar disorder dating back to her 20s. She lives with her husband and two daughters aged 5 and 10 years. They live in a rented two bedroom house on a new housing estate. She has a part-time job in a local pub which supplements the family's main income. She has been married to Andy for just over 10 years following a whirlwind romance and the birth of their first child. The relationship is strained at times because Andy works long hours in his building business. Kate has had a traumatic life: her mother died when she was 8 years old; her father did not cope with her death and began to drink heavily, which caused him to become unpredictable and at times violent. Last year her father died. Following this Kate experienced a depressive phase and attempted suicide. After successfully being treated for this she became hyper-manic, requiring an admission to a mental health ward under the Mental Health Act.*

*Kate is normally a loud a bubbly person who enjoys a good time. However, at the moment Kate is struggling with several issues. Firstly, her 10-year-old daughter is displaying behavioural problems at school—she is still grieving for the loss of her grandfather and is terrified she will lose her mum after her mother's suicide attempt. Secondly, the family are experiencing some financial difficulties with Kate not being able to work for several months and Andy taking time off work to care for the children while Kate was hospitalized. Even though Kate has returned to work, Andy's business has taken a further downturn. Thirdly, Kate was aware that the other mums in the playground were treating her differently and some people who she thought were good friends are now distant with her. Lastly, Kate is experiencing side-effects from her medication. She has gained over one stone in weight and is feeling sedated and unable to concentrate at work. Andy is finding it difficult to understand Kate's presentation and has fears that the children may inherit her illness. All of this has understandably caused relationship strain so that they are arguing, and he says they don't have any fun anymore. Kate is desperate for some help and support.*

---

**Case study 2**

Steven is a 32-year-old man who lives alone in rented accommodation in a deprived area of a major city. His parents are separated and although his mother lives nearby, Steven has little contact with her. He does, however, have a close relationship with his father and sister and although they live further away, they usually manage to see each other several times a month.

Steven has a diagnosis of schizophrenia following a number of psychotic episodes requiring frequent hospital admissions, often under the Mental Health Act. His condition is currently managed through a combination of medication and input from a community mental health nurse. Steven continues to hear voices, which tend to offer a running commentary about him rather than speak directly to him, and which increase in intensity and frequency when he is stressed. For the majority of the time, Steven successfully manages these voices, but they occasionally cause him to feel distressed, frustrated and hopeless. Sometimes Steven also holds unusual beliefs which tend to be of a paranoid nature. During the times that Steven is bothered by these experiences he chooses not to go out or engage in his usual social contacts and activities as he feels too vulnerable.

Steven is a smoker. Normally he smokes approximately 10 cigarettes per day, but would like to reduce this, or give up completely as he is finding it increasingly difficult to afford. Steven also admits to occasionally using alcohol, and previously cannabis, as a way of managing his positive symptoms but again, is aware of the high financial cost of these strategies. He has gained about 10 k in weight following a change in his medication which he is unhappy about.

Steven is not working at the moment and so is in receipt of state benefits. He would like to work but finds motivation a problem. He would also like to move as he finds his current environment intimidating, following an incident where some local youths wrote 'nutter' in spray paint on the wall outside his flat.

Steven has a small circle of friends; some he has known since his school days and some new friends that he has met through the mental health services. He also attends some activities with a voluntary community group, which provide social contact and support. Steven is not currently in a relationship, but hopes one day he will meet someone with whom he can settle down and have a family.

---

## Assessment

Assessment is the systematic collection of data necessary for effective care planning and treatment. It is an ongoing and dynamic process which facilitates the development of a collaborative therapeutic partnership and an understanding of the impact of signs and symptoms on the person's ability to function and quality of life. Throughout the assessment, patients should be allowed the opportunity to 'tell their story' and express their problems as they experience them (Fox and Gamble, 2006).

A variety of assessment tools are available to structure the collection of information (Gamble and Brennan, 2006) and these can be divided into two categories: global assessment tools and clarifying assessment tools. Global assessment takes into account all biopsychosocial needs and includes questions about (DH, 2008a):

- Personal circumstances (including family and/or other carers)
- Psychiatric symptoms and experiences
- Psychological thoughts and behaviours
- Physical health and wellbeing
- Social connections
- Housing circumstances
- Financial circumstances
- Occupation and activity
- Employment and training needs
- Risks and safety
- Drug and alcohol use
- Culture and ethnicity
- Gender and sexuality
- Spiritual needs
- People who depend on you
- Hopes and aspirations
- Strengths.

Information is gathered from a range of perspectives, including the service user, carer and health professional. The process of assessment continues using clarifying tools, which allow a more detailed exploration of specific issues raised during the global assessment. There are many tools available to support the identification and clarification of needs and provide an evidence base for further interventions (Gamble and Brennan, 2006).

Assessment of clients with mental health needs is also considered in the context of the care programme approach (CPA). The CPA is used by specialist mental health services to assess the care needs of, and provide a package of care for, individuals with severe mental illness and a wide range of complex needs (DH, 2008b). It requires a whole-systems approach where services and organizations work together under the coordination of a designated care coordinator (DH, 2008b). The essence of the CPA is a set of principles and values that guide good practice: care is person-centred, collaborative and viewed as a shared responsibility between service user, carer and health and social care professionals.

Both Steven and Kate have diagnoses which fall into the severe mental illness category, and both present with a variety of physical, psychological and social needs requiring a multiagency approach and so, following a comprehensive assessment of their needs, care would be coordinated and managed within the CPA framework.

---

### Reflection

What aspects of assessment do you think are of particular significance for Kate and Steven?

---

## Physical needs and care

The view that individuals with mental health needs have an increased vulnerability to a range of physical conditions is now well established (DH, 2006). Such health risks include endocrinal disorders (diabetes and hyperprolactinemia, which can lead to menstrual disturbances, galactorrhoea and reduced bone mineral density), gastrointestinal (digestive) disorders, respiratory disease and/or infections, cancer (particularly of the breast and colon), hypertension, cardiovascular disease, osteoarthritis, compromised immunity against infection, and metabolic syndrome. Individuals with a mental health problem are twice as likely to die from heart disease than the general population, and people with schizophrenia, psychosis or bipolar disorder are four times more likely to die from respiratory disease and/or infections (Cohen and Hove, 2001; Phelan et al, 2001; Mentality and National Institute for Mental Health in England [NIMHE], 2004). An adult with schizophrenia can expect to live 10 years less than someone without the diagnosis (Disability Rights Commission, 2006).

There are probably a number of interrelated factors that contribute to this situation. It has been demonstrated, for example, that individuals with mental health difficulties have an inadequate intake of fibre and protective antioxidant vitamins owing to a lower consumption of fruit and vegetables, and have higher intakes of saturated fat (Brown et al, 1999). There is also an increased chance that members of this population group have an increased chance of a sedentary lifestyle, particularly in inpatient areas where patients complain of inactivity and boredom (Faulkner, 2005). In the community, formal exercise can be prohibitive because of reduced motivation, cost, accessibility and issues of social inclusion/exclusion, stigma and discrimination. There is a strong link between social disadvantage and poor health (Graham, 2004) — a period of poor mental health and/or diagnosis can result in adverse material conditions, such as unemployment, poverty, debt, homelessness, social rejection and loss of social networks. Such socioeconomic realities can result in an increase in stress levels which, in turn, can have an adverse effect on cholesterol metabolism, blood pressure, blood clotting, platelet aggregability, and immunity against infectious and autoimmune diseases (Mentality and NIMHE, 2004). There is also a strong association between mental health diagnosis and higher rates of alcohol and substance use/misuse (Mentality and NIMHE, 2004), and raised rates of smoking (Etter et al, 2004). It is estimated that 61% of individuals with schizophrenia and 46% of individuals with bipolar disorder are smokers compared with 33% of the general population (Disability Rights Commission, 2006).

Medication, while of benefit for a range of signs and symptoms, can also contribute negatively to the overall health of an individual. Weight gain is a known side-effect of most psychotropic medications, including antipsychotics, antidepressants and mood stabilizers (Stahl, 2000; Pulzer 2006), which is a likely factor contributing to high levels of obesity (Fagiolini et al, 2008) — it is estimated that 33% of individuals with schizophrenia and 30% of individuals with bipolar disorder are obese compared with 21% of the general population (Disability Rights Comission, 2006). Hyperglycaemia, abdominal obesity, reduced high-density lipoprotein (HDL) cholesterol, raised triglyceride and raised blood pressure (known collectively as metabolic syndrome) can also be a consequence of the second generation, or atypical, antipsychotics leading to an increased risk of diabetes, a sudden cardiac event, or stroke (Jones and Jones, 2008).

Health service provision may also have an inadvertent adverse effect on the physical health of this group of individuals. It has been suggested that mental health nurses often lack the skills and confidence to deal adequately with service users' physical health needs or too frequently ascribe psychological causes to the signs and symptoms of physical conditions. Non-mental health trained staff often feel ill-equipped and uncomfortable dealing with mental health issues and therefore fail to successfully engage with patients (Phelan, 2001; DH, 2005). There is also evidence to suggest that there is poor uptake of routine screening within this patient group, despite visiting their GPs more frequently than other patients (Mentality and NIMHE, 2004).

An awareness and knowledge of the health risks of individuals with long-term mental health needs is the first step in improving the physical health of such individuals, as once these issues are acknowledged, then the care team can set about introducing preventive and protective strategies. Just the fact that Kate and Steven both have diagnoses consistent with what are considered long-term, or enduring, mental health problems makes them more vulnerable to developing one or more of the physical conditions described. Both Kate and Steven have experienced significant increases in weight gain which, in addition to any psychological impact, increases the risk of coronary heart disease, diabetes, hypertension, gall bladder disease, and certain cancers (Tardieu et al, 2003). They have both been prescribed medication to help manage the distressing symptoms of their presentations, and both experience increased levels of stress associated with aspects of their mental health issues. Steven tends to use alcohol and cannabis as a way of managing this stress and is also a regular smoker.

One of the most important aspects of managing the physical health care of people like Kate and Steven is successful team working and a clear and documented care plan which details who is responsible for what. There is often confusion between the responsibilities of the primary care team and secondary care services, particularly when individuals with known mental health needs are cared for in the community. The shared CPA documentation should facilitate effective communication and correspondence between all individuals involved in care management and delivery, and formal sharing of information should occur annually (DH, 2008b).

One of the most consistent recommendations found in the literature is the need for an annual health check (DH, 2006). This principle is also included in the new General Medical Services (nGMS) contract in England (NHS Employers, 2005), which requires GPs to develop a register of all individuals with schizophrenia and bipolar disorder to enable the annual health check to be targeted at this group. The annual health check should, ideally, be an opportunity to both gather and offer information, and should include an assessment of blood pressure, pulse, height and weight, to calculate body mass index (BMI), waist measurement, current medication and any existing physical illnesses and/or conditions. Lifestyle factors such as diet, exercise, alcohol and drug use, sexual behaviour and smoking should also be explored alongside any family history, particularly of cardiovascular disease and diabetes. A full blood count and liver function test is also recommended to establish the individual's ability to metabolize prescribed medication (Jones and Jones, 2008), as are blood tests to establish thyroid function, lipids, glucose and prolactin levels. Some medications such as lithium, a mood stabilizing drug, and clozapine, a second generation anti-psychotic, also require specialist blood monitoring. Owing to the cardiotoxicity of some psychotropic medication, an electrocardiogram might also be indicated. Preventive measures such as cervical smears, breast and prostate screening, bone density measurement, and the flu vaccination should also be considered alongside a review of other physical health needs such as dentistry, chiropody, sexual health, sight and hearing. Once a full assessment of physical need has been accomplished then further interventions can be implemented around medication management, diet, exercise and smoking cessation.

In terms of medication management, it is important to consider psychotropic medication in the context of the physical health assessment to ensure the choice of psychiatric medication does not further compromise the individual's physical health. This can be achieved through discussions between the service user, the prescriber and any other professionals or carers. Not only will this improve physical health outcomes, it is also likely to have a positive impact on concordance (Jones and Jones, 2008).

As weight gain is one of the most troubling side-effects of psychotropic medication (Dean et al, 2001), and poses the biggest risk to physical health, it is essential to identify strategies to help Steven and Kate reduce their body weight, as even a 5% reduction in weight significantly improves morbidity and mortality rates (Thomas, 2005). This can be achieved using interventions that focus on lifestyle choices. Although this can be difficult in a population group that is often socioeconomically compromised, small changes can still have a beneficial effect on physical health outcomes. General dietary advice should be routinely initiated (British Nutrition Foundation, 2007). Organizations such as Rethink and the Mental Health Foundation produce useful information on how to achieve a balanced diet within limited resources. Lifestyle or healthy living groups (Smith et al, 2007) are also increasingly available in both primary and secondary care services, and not only provide useful advice and monitoring regarding positive health choices, but also provide a source of support and social contact.

Owing to the huge and varied benefits of increased activity levels, such as improving physical and mental health outcomes, increasing self-esteem and social contact, it has been suggested that clinicians should consider physical activity as a routine aspect of care (DH, 2006). Factors that influence the success of an achievable and sustainable exercise programme include ensuring the activity is culturally-sensitive and tailored to individual needs (Richardson et al, 2005), avoiding unrealistic expectations, setting small incremental increases and goals, and providing supportive leadership with positive feedback and reinforcement. Walking can also provide a low-cost alternative to structured programmes and can be integrated into daily schedules.

Guidelines from the National Institute for Health and Clinical Excellence (NICE) (2006) on smoking recommend that all people who smoke should be asked how interested they are in quitting (cessation). Steven has expressed a desire to reduce his smoking habit, and therefore help and support to help him achieve this goal should be offered. Smoking cessation guidelines for health professionals recommend the 'four As' approach: ask, advise, assist, and arrange (Robson and Gray, 2005). Timing should also be considered as breaking the habit might not be appropriate when symptoms are active. Evidence suggests that a combination of approaches achieves the greatest success (Bradshaw et al, 2005), for example individual and/or group therapy/support with nicotine replacement seem to have a better long-term outcome than a singular approach. A review of medication might also be advisable as it appears that abstinence rates are higher in individuals who are prescribed atypical antipsychotic medication.

However, the success of all these interventions ultimately depends on the success of the therapeutic relationship. Interventions and strategies should be patient-centred and approached collaboratively. Any change in lifestyle, no matter how positive the outcome, involves costs as well as benefits. It is therefore essential that this is acknowledged and included in the overall care package.

---

### Reflection

• What do you think are the greatest physical health risks for Kate and Steven?
• How might you help them reduce these risks?

---

## Psychological needs and care

The meeting of psychological need is often a neglected area of clinical practice. While deficiencies in both physical and social care are often more visible to the service provider and society, the provision of care to meet psychological need is also paramount.

It is well established that being identified as having an 'enduring' or 'serious mental illness' attracts societal stigma leading to the experience of discrimination and service inequality (Corrigan et al, 2004). Diagnoses such as schizophrenia and bipolar disorder attract public misunderstanding and fear, which are contributory factors in sufferers often experiencing limited access to social networks and forms of social support (Bebbington and Kuipers, 2008). From a psychological perspective, the diagnostic label itself can be sufficient to cause severe damage to the individual's self-esteem and self-image, and this can be exacerbated by continual exposure to the negative effects of discrimination that so many people with long-term mental health problems experience (Wahl, 1999).

Viewing major mental illnesses, such as schizophrenia and bipolar affective disorder, from the stress–vulnerability perspective accommodates a broad, flexible and patient-centred approach that allows for the biological, psychological and social influences to be considered with equal merit in terms of causation and in relation to risk and relapse (Clements and Turpin, 1992).

Zubin and Spring (1977: 109) described a stress–vulnerability model in which 'each of us is endowed with a degree of vulnerability that under suitable circumstances will express itself in an episode of schizophrenic illness. Some people have high degrees of vulnerability that result in them developing symptoms of illness, while others have low vulnerability (Brennan, 2006). Describing both the concepts of in-born and acquired vulnerability, Zubin and Spring (1977) outlined a process whereby stressful events test an individual's 'adaptive capacities', and if compromised, could result in illness. The severity of the stress is determined by the individual's own perception of it.

Nuechterlein (1987) extended the model of stress–vulnerability further to incorporate personal and environmental protectors, such as a range of developed coping responses and psychosocial interventions, which may be successful in reducing an individual's susceptibility to environmental stress.

Adopting a stress–vulnerability framework would allow service providers, and both Kate and Steven, to share some common ground on which to examine their problems and collaboratively plan and deliver care.

The importance of a strongly rooted and secure sense of self to good mental health cannot be underestimated and if we are fortunate enough to experience a secure and loving upbringing, the less likely we will be excessively influenced by external factors and feedback, however negative (Watkins, 2007). For both Steven and Kate, the experience of severe mental ill-health may compromise their sense of self and result in their being personally vulnerable.

Steven has been exposed to stigmatizing abuse, is intimidated in his current living environment, has a limited social network and social support, and is undergoing a negative change in body image—all of which can impact negatively on his self-esteem.

Kate also feels that her illness has stigmatized her and she is undergoing an unwanted change in body shape, both of which can further compromise an already fragile self-esteem.

Therapeutic interventions with both Kate and Steven, as well as offering help and support to deal with the effects of social exclusion, stigma and unwanted weight gain, would need to focus on assisting them to develop a positive sense of self accompanied by strategies to help them maintain this when faced with crisis and stress (Lloyd and King, 2007).

The issues of 'loss' and 'change' are important to consider when examining the effects of long-term mental ill-health. Many sufferers describe both sadness and anger for the disruption that illness has caused to their lives and may need help to rediscover their potential and redefine their goals, hopes and aspirations for life within the context of adapting to their illness (Watkins, 2007).

Carers will often need support to cope with what they perceive as a 'loss' of their loved one, and to adjust to the changes in the person with the illness. Both Steven, Kate and their families may benefit from targeted therapeutic approaches that as well as providing much needed education about the illness, would also provide the opportunity to explore loss, change and adjustment (Kuipers et al, 2002).

Kate's children, in particular, may struggle to cope with the perceived loss of their mother and the effects of her illness on their lives, and there is a proven link between parental mental ill-health and subsequent child distress and dysfunction (Royal College of Psychiatrists, 2002). Kate and her family, having so recently been affected by the death of a close relative, also have specific needs that may require specialist bereavement counselling aimed at helping them cope with one of life's most enduring stressors.

Long-term conditions such as schizophrenia and bipolar mood disorder can affect the cognitive functioning of the individual in a variety of ways. The major symptoms can disturb perception, thought and mood, and it is frequently these that often provide the main focus for diagnosis and the target for subsequent 'treatment' from health professionals (Mills et al, 2006). However, for the person experiencing the illness, the way it makes him/her 'feel' and the effects that it has on this/her ability to think, is a significant issue (Watkins, 1996).

Perceptual disturbances, most commonly 'hearing voices' and holding unusual beliefs (also referred to as 'delusions'), can be both frightening and distressing experiences, and can be disruptive to the individual's attempts to engage with aspects of daily living. While not universally malevolent or threatening, a significant percentage of sufferers report experiences in which their personal safety or integrity feels compromised (Nyani and David, 1979). Consequently, living in a personal environment in which you perceive your safety cannot be guaranteed is particularly stressful. As well helping to support the development of personal psychological safety, therapeutic interventions would need to acknowledge existing strengths, coping strategies, explore a range of possible psychosocial interventions, and be aware of potential risk issues.

The impact of cognitive blunting, whether this is a consequence of the sedative effects of neuroleptic medication or results from the collection of 'negative' symptoms that accompany schizophrenia (loss of motivation, social withdrawal and slowed thinking), can severely disrupt the ability to function. It would appear that for both Kate and Steven, levels of cognitive functioning have been affected by their illness and subsequent treatment, and adopting a collaborative approach to managing medication could enhance concordance with the regimen and achieve maximum efficacy with minimum side-effects (Gray, 2002).

Learning to regain those aspects of cognitive functioning that can be blunted by the effects of long-term illness requires a gentle approach that is both patient and persistent, and which encourages the slow and steady progress towards 'recovery' (Mills et al, 2006; Watkins, 2007).

---

### Reflection

- Identify some possible stressors that could have an impact on Steven and Kate's psychological wellbeing
- What interventions might you suggest to reduce their vulnerability to the effects of stress?

---

## Social needs and care

Individuals with mental health difficulties often experience a variety of social difficulties. There is evidence to suggest that individuals within this group, particularly those with a psychotic disorder, are more likely to have not completed their education, be unemployed, have a reduced income, incur debt and have difficulty paying bills, experience insecurity with accommodation owing to financial problems, to be single, divorced or separated, and have a small primary support group of three or fewer people (DH, 2002). In addition, they are also more likely to experience difficulties with activities of daily living such as personal care, using transport, managing medical care, household activities, practical activities, and managing money (DH, 2002).

Although some individuals blame the illness itself (Rethink et al, 2008), many of these social difficulties are often bound up with issues of stigma, discrimination and social exclusion. Users of mental health services often find themselves 'among the most unequal, disenfranchised, disempowered and excluded members' of our communities (Mentality and NIMHE, 2004). Stigma and discrimination can manifest in a variety of ways. Although there is an acknowledgement that stigma and discrimination are multilayered and complex problems, the 2008 'Stigma Shout' survey found that stigma prevents people from seeking help, delays treatment, impairs recovery, causes isolation, excludes people from day-to-day activities, and hinders employment (Rethink et al, 2008). Respondents felt that stigma and discrimination had a negative impact on several areas of their lives including employment, new and existing friendships, being able to join groups and take part in activities within the community, confidence to get out and about, the ability to disclose mental health issues, and the ability to challenge professionals (Rethink et al, 2008). Both Steven and Kate are experiencing several of the issues highlighted by this research. Both live in rented accommodation, experience reduced income and financial restriction, feel socially isolated and alienated, and feel rejected and, in Steven's case, intimidated by their community. In addition, Steven is single, has a reduced primary support group, lives in an economically-deprived area and is unemployed. Challenging stigma and discrimination and promoting social inclusion requires the 'whole systems', collaborative approach endorsed within the CPA framework, and needs systematic and strategic social and community support.

Although the average paid employment rate for individuals with a mental health problem is lower than in any other disadvantaged group, with only 22% being in paid employment or full-time education (Healthcare Commission, 2008) compared with 74.2% of the average UK employment rate (Office for National Statistics [ONS], 2008), the majority of people with mental health problems consistently say they want to work (Sainsbury Centre for Mental Health, 2009). In recognition that occupation improves physical and mental health, is effective in improving social inclusion (National Social Inclusion Programme [NSIP], 2009), and has a positive impact on socioeconomic circumstances, there are a growing number of initiatives to improve employment rates within this group.

The NSIP has responded to the Government's action plan on social exclusion (Cabinet Office, 2006) by developing regional employment teams to promote partnership working between key employment organizations and raise awareness of mental health in the workplace, in addition to supporting the mental health first aid scheme which trains individuals to care for someone experiencing a mental health problem before professional help is sought. Another example is the Individual Placement and Support (IPS) scheme, which offers intensive individual support and rapid job search followed by placement in paid employment and unlimited work-based support for both the employer and the employee (Sainsbury Centre for Mental Health, 2009). The Trade Union Congress (TUC) (2008) has also published practical guidance to improve the recruitment, retention and fair treatment of service users within the workplace and suggests practical measures such as more flexible working hours, offering someone a 'workplace buddy', changing someone's duties if they become unwell, and keeping in regular supportive contact during periods of sick leave.

Another measure introduced to promote social inclusion is the introduction of individual budgets designed to give patients greater choice and control over their social needs. Although only a pilot scheme at the time of writing, the evaluation with regard to mental health service users appears positive (Glendinning et al, 2008), and indicates that participants have used the payments to purchase a range of services including personal care, domestic help, and social, leisure and educational activities (Allen, 2008). This therefore allows service users to participate 'in society in ways more acceptable to them than those offered by existing day or other services' (Allen, 2008), to feel more in control of their daily lives, and report a significantly higher quality of life (Glendinning et al, 2008).

Such practical measures are also being underpinned by the launch of a four-year campaign to reduce the stigma and discrimination of mental health in England. With a similar agenda to the 'See Me' campaign in Scotland (See Me Alliance, 2008), 'Time to Change' (Mental Health Media et al, 2008) aims to publically challenge attitudes towards mental health and reduce discrimination. This will be achieved through a variety of projects, covering social marketing, physical activity, anti-stigma training, community action, and legal issues.

---

### Reflection

- In what ways are the issues of stigma, discrimination and social exclusion affecting the lives of Kate and Steven?
- What action might you take to help them address these issues?

---

## Conclusion

The signs and symptoms of a long-term mental health condition can, in themselves, be disabling in a variety of ways; however, the lived experience beyond the label or diagnosis includes a range of complex physical, psychological and social needs, as demonstrated through the examples of Steven and Kate. In order to effectively identify and meet these needs, a person-centred, collaborative and comprehensive assessment involving a range of health and social care professionals is paramount.

Successful care delivery requires a coordinated approach, based on good communication and team-working, which aims to enable individuals like

Steven and Kate to work towards 'recovery', meet their goals, and achieve their full potential.

Allen D (2008) Putting people back in control. *Ment Health Pract* **12**(4): 6

Bebbington P, Kuipers E (2008) Psychosocial factors. In: Mueser KT, Jeste DV. eds, *Clinical Handbook of Schizophrenia*. The Guilford Press, New York

Bradshaw T, Lovell K, Harris N (2005) Healthy living interventions with schizophrenia: a systematic review. *J Adv Nurs* **49**(6): 634–54

British Nutrition Foundation (2007) Heart Disease and Stroke. British Nutrition Foundation, London

Brennan G (2006) Stress vulnerability model of serious mental illness. In: Gamble C, Brennan G. eds, *Working with Serious Mental Illness: a manual for clinical practice*. 2nd edn. Elsevier Ltd, Philadelphia

Brown S, Birtwistle J, Roe L, Thompson C (1999) The unhealthy lifestyle of people with schizophrenia. *Psychol Med* **29**(3): 697–701

Cabinet Office (2006) Reaching Out: An Action Plan on Social Exclusion. http://tinyurl. com/5sorzn (accessed 10 November 2009)

Clements K, Turpin G (1992) Vulnerability models and schizophrenia: the assessment and prediction of relapse. In: Birchwood M, Tarrier N. eds, *Innovations in the Psychological Management of Schizophrenia: Assessment, treatment and services*. John Wiley, Chichester

Cohen A, Hove M (2001) *Physical Health of People with Severe Mental Illness: a training pack for GP educators*. The Sainsbury Centre for Mental Health, London

Corrigan P, Markowitz F, Watson A (2004) Structural levels of mental illness, stigma and discrimination. *Schizophr Bull* **30**(3): 481–91

Dean J, Todd G, Morrow H, Sheldon K (2001) 'Mum, I used to be good looking ... look at me now'. The physical health needs of adults with mental health problems: the perspectives of users, carers and front-line staff. *Int J Ment Health Promot* **3**(4): 16–24

DH (1999) *A National Service Framework for Mental Health: Modern Standards and Service Models*. DH, London. ref: 1999

DH (2002) *The social and economic circumstances of adults with mental disorders*. DH, London. ref: 2002

DH (2005) *Meeting the physical needs of individuals with mental health problems and the mental health needs of individuals cared for in general health sectors: advice from the Standing Nursing and Midwifery Advisory Committee (SNMAC)*. DH, London

DH (2006) *Choosing Health: Supporting the physical needs of people with severe mental illness—commissioning framework*. DH, London. ref: 6757

DH (2008a) Making the CPA work for you: It is not how you fit into services, It is about how services fit with you. http://tinyurl.com/y9u832v (accessed 10 November 2009)

DH (2008b) *Refocusing the Care Programme Approach: policy and positive practice guidance*. DH, London. ref: 9148

Disability Rights Commission (2006) *Equal Treatment: Closing the Gap*. Disability Rights Commission, Stratford on Avon

Engel G (1977) The need for a new medical model: a challenge for biomedicine. *Science* **196**(4286): 129–36

Etter M, Mohr S, Garin C, Etter JF (2004) Stages of change in smokers with schizophrenia or schizoaffective disorder and in the general population. *Schizophr Bull* **30**(2): 459–68

Fagiolini A, Chengappa KNR, Soreca I, Chang J (2008) Bipolar disorder and the metabolic syndrome: causal factors, psychiatric outcomes and economic burden. *CNS Drugs* **22**(8): 655–69

Faulkner G (2005) Exercise as an adjunct treatment for schizophrenia. In: Faulkner G, Taylor A. eds, *Exercise, Health and Mental Health: emerging relationships*. Routledge, Abingdon

Fox J, Gamble C (2006) Consolidating the assessment process: the semi-structured interview. In: Gamble C, Brennan G. eds, *Working with Serious Mental Illness: A Manual for Clinical Practice*. 2nd edn. Elsevier, London

Gamble C, Brennan G (2006) Assessments: a rationale for choosing and using. In: Gamble C, Brennan G. eds, *Working with Serious Mental Illness: a manual for clinical practice*. 2nd edn. Elsevier Ltd. Philiadelphia

Glendinning C, Challis D, Fernandez J et al (2008) Evaluation of the Individual Budgets Pilot Progreamme: Final Report. http://php.york.ac.uk/inst/spru/pubs/1119/ (accessed 10 November 2009)

Graham H (2004) Socio-economic Inequalities in Health in the UK: evidence on patterns and determinants. http://tinyurl.com/yjsrw45 (accessed 10 November 2009)

Gray R (2002) Medication management for people with a diagnosis of schizophrenia. *Nurs Times* **98**(47): 38–40

Healthcare Commission (2008) *Mental Health Service Users Survey*. Healthcare Commission, London

Jones M, Jones A (2008) The effect of antipsychotic medication on metabolic syndrome. *Nurs Stand* **22**(48): 43–8

Kuipers E, Leff J, Lam D (2002) *Family work for schizophrenia: A practical guide*. 2nd edn. Gaskell, London

Lloyd C, King R (2007) Early intervention, relapse prevention and promotion of healthy lifestyles. In: King R, Lloyd C, Meehan T. eds, *Handbook of Psychosocial Rehabilitation*. Blackwell, London

Mental Health Media, Mind, Rethink, Institute of Psychiatry (2008) Time to Change. www.time-to-change.org.uk (accessed 10 November 2009)

Mentality and National Institute of Mental Health in England (2004) *Healthy Body Healthy Mind: promoting healthy living for people who experience mental health problems.* Mentality and NIMHE, London

Mills J, Kerr S, Goldspink S (2006) Dealing with blankness and deadness. In: Gamble C, Brennan G. eds, *Working with Serious Mental Illness: A Manual for Clinical Practice.* 2nd edn. Elsevier, London

National Social Inclusion Programme (2009) *Vision and Progress: social inclusion and mental health.* NSIP, London

NHS Employers (2005) *Investing in General Practice: Revisions to the General Medical Service Contract for 2006–2007 in England.* NHS Employers, London

NICE (2006) Brief interventions and referral for smoking cessation in primary care and other settings. http://guidance.nice.org.uk/PH1 (accessed 10 November 2009)

Nuechterlein K (1987) Vulnerability models for schizophrenia: state of the art. In: Hafner H, Gattaz W, Janarzik W. eds, *Search for the Causes of Schizophrenia.* Springer, Berline

Nyani T, David A (1979) The auditory hallucination: a phenomenological survey. *Psychol Med* **26**: 177–89

Office for National Statistics (2008) *Labour Force Survey: National and Regional Indicators August–October 2008.* ONS, London

Phelan M, Stradins L, Morrison S (2001) Physical health of people with severe mental illness. *BMJ* **322**(7284): 434–4

Pulzer M (2006) Metabolic syndrome and anti-psychotic drugs. *Ment Health Nurs* **26**(6): 17–9

Rethink, Mind, Mental Health Media (2008) *Stigma Shout: service user and carer experiences of stigma and discrimination.* Rethink, London

Richardson CR, Faulkner G, McDevitt J et al (2005) Integrating physical activity into mental health services for persons with serious mental illness. *Psychiatr Serv* **56**(3): 324–31

Robson D, Gray R (2005) Can we help people with schizophrenia stop smoking? *Ment Health Pract* **9**(4): 15–8

Royal College of Psychiatrists (2002) *Patients as parents: Addressing the needs, including safety, of children whose parents are mentally ill.* CR105. Royal College of Psychiatrists, London

Royal College of Psychiatrists (2004) *Schizophrenia.* Royal College of Psychiatrists, London

Royal College of Psychiatrists (2007) *Bipolar Disorder.* Royal College of Psychiatrists, London

Sainsbury Centre for Mental Health (2009) *Doing What Works: Individual Placement Support into Employment Briefing.* Sainsbury Centre for Mental Health, London

See Me (2008) *See Me National Plan 2008–2011.* See Me Alliance, Leith

Smith S, Yeomans D, Bushe C et al (2007) A well-being programme in severe mental illness. Baseline findings in a UK cohort. *Int J Clin Pract* **61**(12): 1971–8

Stahl SM (2000) *Essential Psychopharmacology: neuroscientific basis and practical applications.* 2nd edn. Cambridge University Press, Cambridge

Tardieu S, Micallef J. Gentile S, Blin O (2003) Weight gain profiles of new anti-psychotics: public health consequences. *Obes Rev* **4**(3): 129–38

Thomas PR (2005) *Weighing the pptions: criteria for evaluating weight-management programs.* National Academy Press, Washington DC

Trades Union Congress (2008) Representing and supporting members with mental health problems at work: Guidance for trade union representatives. www.tuc.org.uk/extras/mentalhealth.pdf (accessed 10 November 2009)

Wahl OF (1999) Mental health consumers' experience of stigma. *Schizophr Bull* **25**(3): 467–78

Watkins J (1996) *Living with schizophrenia: an holistic approach to understanding, preventing and recovering from negative symptoms.* Hill of Content, Australia

Watkins P (2007) *Recovery: A Guide for Mental Health Practitioners.* Churchill Livingstone, China

World Health Organization (1992) International Classification of Diseases (ICD). www.who.int/classifications/icd/en (accessed 10 November 2009)

Zubin J, Spring B (1977) Vulnerability—a new view of schizophrenia. *J Abnorm Psychol* **86**(2): 103–66

# Further information

*Mental Health First Aid England: www.mentalhealthfirstaid.csip.org.uk*

*Shift: www.shift.org.uk*

*Time to change: www.time-to-change.org.uk*

# CHAPTER 12

# The weigh forward

*Janice Strefford and Jasmin Amoroso*

*This chapter explores the issue of obesity. The authors demonstrate how, using a proactive approach, effective strategies to target and manage obesity can be introduced. The Weigh Forward programme is an ongoing project that is currently being developed. This account looks at the development and planning stages of the project.*

Obesity has long been associated with the development of many long-term conditions and is directly related to increased mortality and reduced life expectancy (Must et al, 1999). Obesity is linked to 9000 premature deaths per year in England, and reduces life expectancy by an average of nine years. Obesity also has considerable cost implications; the NHS spends approximately £1 billion per year on the condition (Department of Health [DH], 2007). Furthermore, obesity incurs a further £2.3–2.6 billion per year to our total economy, for example by causing other long-term conditions that incur protracted treatment costs and increased social support and disability allowance for the social services budget, from loss of time or cessation of work with associated illnesses (Counterweight, 2005a). Wanless estimated that if the current trend continues, the cost to the total economy could rise to £3.6 billion per year by 2010 (DH, 2007).

Tackling obesity is a Government-wide priority (DH, 2009), supported by *Healthy Weight, Healthy Lives: A Cross-Government Strategy for England* (DH, 2008a). A total of £372 million has been allocated to implement the strategy, which identifies how the Government will enable everyone in society to maintain a healthy weight (DH, 2009).

This chapter discusses the development of a strategy for tackling familial obesity. It explores the development of a weight management programme, 'Weigh Forward', in rural Leicestershire. Reading this chapter and reflecting on your own experiences should enable you to meet the following learning outcomes:

- Identify the health risks associated with obesity
- Identify the benefits of proactively managing obesity in primary care
- Examine the process of service development.

## Background

The practice population in this rural area of Leicestershire predominantly comprises white people. At the time of writing, the practice had 683 people on the obesity register out of nearly 10 000 patients registered at the practice—7% of the total practice population. However, experience shows that some people refuse to be weighed, and some people are too heavy for the 200 kg scales, so the number of obese patients is probably far higher. In line with Government policy, the practice has been targeting obesity; practice audit has shown that this has had varying degrees of success. The initiative for the 'Weigh Forward' programme was conceived because one area where success had been limited was with children, and especially when obesity was prevalent within their families.

When considering the families within which obesity was prevalent, it was recognized that there was a commonality of undesirable lifestyle behaviour patterns. These are being passed through the family to each generation, and could result in the perpetuation of associated lifestyle diseases. It was agreed that it would be valuable to develop a service comprising weight management courses for family groups. Key stages from the planning and evaluation cycle were used to structure the action plan (Ewles and Simnett, 2003) (*Table 12.1*).

---

**Table 12.1 Key stages for planning and evaluation of health promotion**

1. Identify needs and priorities
2. Set aims and objectives
3. Determine best method to achieve aims
4. Identify available and required resources
5. Plan methods of evaluation
6. Set action plan
7. Implementation of action plan (evaluation should be ongoing throughout the process)

From: Ewles and Simnett (2003)

---

# Identifying needs and priorities

The first consideration, before targeting efforts, was to review whether familial obesity should actually be prioritized. Obesity occurs when a person puts on weight to the point that it seriously endangers health. This is caused by a combination of eating too many calories and not taking enough exercise. However, for most people it is reversible through a change in lifestyle. This makes it worth prioritizing. Additionally, obesity is a lifestyle disease that increases risk of many long-term conditions, for example 58% of type 2 diabetes and 21% of heart disease incidence can be linked to obesity (DH, 2007).

Obesity is currently categorized using a body mass index (BMI) measurement ($kg/m^2$):

- Overweight = BMI of 25–29.9
- Obesity = BMI of more than 30
- Morbid obesity = BMI of more than 40
- Malignant obesity = BMI of more than 50.

There is more variation in how 'overweight' and 'obesity' are defined in children. However, childhood is a time of development, and BMI is not a static measurement. Age and gender-specific BMI centile charts, adjusted for growth, have been designed by the Child Growth Foundation (National Obesity Forum, 2009a).

Worldwide, obesity levels have been steadily rising for a number of years. Obesity levels have tripled in England since 1980, with no sign of this upward trend coming to a halt (DH, 2008a). Incidence continues to rise in England: one in four adults is obese; over half of women and approximately two thirds of men are overweight or obese; and if current trends continue, 28% women and 33% men will be obese by 2010 (Zaninotto et al, 2006).

Obesity causes approximately 18 million sick days and 30 000 deaths in England every year. Most obese people develop some related physical symptoms by the age of 40 years (National Prescribing Centre, 2009). As a result of continuing obesity, the majority of people proceed to develop diseases that require medical intervention by the age of 60 years (National Prescribing Centre, 2009). Mortality figures indicate that life expectancy is reduced on average by nine years as a result of obesity (National Audit Office [NAO], 2001).

With regard to children, surveillance from 2007/08 shows that approximately 31% of boys and 30% of girls are overweight or obese (NHS Information Centre, 2008). A year-on-year rise in obesity among children under 11 years was predicted by 2010 (Zaninotto et al, 2006). Furthermore, the Government's scientific expert committee, the Foresight team, predicts that by 2050, 55% of boys and 70% of girls could be overweight or obese (Foresight, 2007). The authors recognized that many children in the practice will go on to have their own children. If they perpetuate their familial patterns of behaviour, they will very likely be the parents and grandparents of those in the predicted Foresight group by 2050.

This evidence was compelling; tackling obesity is a confirmed national health priority, which is being addressed with vigorous political will. The authors felt it was essential to develop a strategy that would help to break the cycle of unhealthy behaviours within obese families. However, it is necessary to ensure that targeting familial obesity, rather than working with individuals, is worthwhile. The DH (2008a) showed that targeting health advice at families, and helping them to raise fitness levels and eat more healthily, is more effective than targeting adults or children in isolation. Organizations such as the National Obesity Forum (2009a) and MEND (2009) support familial work.

The families who were initially targeted were those in which several family members were obese, and in which it was identified that children, parents and grandparents share a lifestyle of poor diet and little or no exercise. The authors felt that this would be beneficial to the whole family, not just the children, because being overweight or obese increases the risk of developing health problems in adulthood. It is likely that older family members will already have such health problems.

Having recognized that obesity increases the risk of many long-term conditions, related disease risks were examined (Weight Control Information Network, 2007; Centers for Disease Control and Prevention, 2009; National Obesity Forum, 2009b):

- Premature death—obese people have a 50–100% increased risk of premature death from all causes, compared to individuals with a healthy weight
- Immune system—more likely to die from seasonal influenza
- Heart—arrhythmia, angina, heart attack and heart failure
- Blood pressure—hypertension
- Blood lipids—e.g. high total cholesterol, high triglycerides
- Brain—stroke and dementia
- Pancreas—insulin resistance and diabetes
- Lungs—asthma and other breathing difficulties
- Oesophagus and stomach—gastric-oesophageal reflux disease (GORD)
- Gall bladder—gall stones
- Liver—non-alcoholic fatty liver disease/cirrhosis
- Colon—cancer

---

**Table 12.2 Benefits of 10% reduction in body weight**

**Blood pressure**
Systolic and diastolic fall of approximately 10 mmHg
in hypertensive patients

**Diabetes**
40–60% fall in diabetes incidence
30% increase in insulin sensitivity
Up to 50% fall in fasting glucose for newly diagnosed patients
30% fall in fasting blood glucose

**Lipids**
10% fall in total cholesterol
15% fall in low-density lipoprotein
30% fall in triglycerides
8% increase in high-density lipoprotein

**Mortality**
20% fall in all-cause mortality
30% fall in diabetes-related deaths
40% fall in obesity-related deaths

From: National Audit Office (2001); Haslam et al (2006); Department of Health (2007)

---

- Spine—lumbar pain
- Ovaries—menstrual disorders, infertility and polycystic ovaries
- Uterus—cancer
- Bladder—incontinence
- Breasts—cancer
- Knees—increased risk of arthritis by 35% for every 11 lb of extra weight
- Wellbeing—sleep apnoea
- Social and psychological problems, such as depression, prejudice, discrimination, stigmatization and low self-esteem.

Having identified the risks of obesity, the authors considered the potential benefits of weight loss. Maintaining a healthy weight reduces the risk of all comorbidities. Haslam et al (2006) reported more specific metabolic and vascular benefits of losing 10% of body weight (*Table 12.2*).

The NAO (2001) has predicted that one million fewer obese people in the UK could lead to around 15 000 fewer people with coronary heart disease, 34 000 fewer people developing type 2 diabetes, and 99 000 fewer people with high blood pressure (DH, 2007).

Evaluation of the evidence provided adequate information to prioritize service development. This enabled the advancement of list of long-term benefits that the programme hoped to achieve, which were then formalized as the desired outcomes of the project.

## Aims

The overall aims of the Weigh Forward project are to provide a sustainable programme of weight management courses for family groups. To facilitate this aim, specific objectives to meet 'SMART' criteria, as recommended by the NHS Modernisation Agency (2005), were planned:

S   Specific, by being relevant to this client group
M   Measurable, by enabling patients and clinicians to measure results
A   Achievable, by tailoring advice to involve acceptable lifestyle modifications for each family
R   Realistic, by using services which are locally available and acceptable
T   Timely, by setting deadlines and by offering an appropriate number of course sessions at acceptable times.

## Objectives

- To inform key stakeholders, seeking approval and funding
- To identify the families most at risk of obesity and its complications
- To develop course and action plans
- To identify human, material and financial resources
- To develop an evaluation strategy
- To use the evaluation findings to develop a maintenance programme at the end of the intensive programmes

## Outcomes

- To promote reduction in familial obesity through the adoption of healthier lifestyles, focusing on improved diet and increased exercise
- To raise awareness of the health issues relating to obesity
- To improve families' knowledge of strategies to improve lifestyle using a variety of interventions
- To empower families to make healthier lifestyle choices

- To facilitate changes in attitudes and behaviour
- To bring about social change, albeit at a local level.

## Achieving the objectives

### Objective 1

Approval was paramount to gain permission to proceed; therefore, this was the primary consideration. A proposal was presented to the GPs and the practice manager, which received positive approval. Next, the proposal was submitted to the local primary care trust (PCT). An introduction was written to demonstrate that the service would meet stated PCT goals and measures, and was subsequently approved to include funding.

### Objective 2

To identify the families at highest risk, the authors accessed the local obesity register, which was compiled to meet Quality and Outcomes Framework (QOF) Indicator OB1 (DH, 2005). Obese children were identified and the authors reflected on which ones were members of the type of families that the programme aimed to target. The weight records of family members were reviewed to confirm these reflections.

### Objective 3

To develop the course plan, the authors used experiences of health promotion groups. As obesity comes about when the intake of food exceeds the energy exerted, it was agreed that the service should look at patient lifestyles holistically. The involvement of multidisciplinary and multiagency colleagues in the service, particularly in the delivery of sessions, would provide a range of interventions, resulting in a comprehensive package that would bring different dimensions to the course (Scottish Intercollegiate Guidelines Network [SIGN], 2003). The authors felt that this eclectic approach would facilitate the range of choices being offered. This, in turn, should meet the different learning styles of patients, thereby increasing the chance of offering something to suit everyone. The course was designed to include all family members, and also—to maximize potential—to involve the wider community as much as possible. During each session, a variety of styles and incentives were planned. This maximizes the opportunity for each person to explore their own health beliefs and challenge them. The intended aim is to improve knowledge, thereby helping to change attitudes and behaviour.

To raise awareness of obesity as a health problem, a variety of media, drawing on national and local initiatives, such as national radio and TV, 'change4life' materials (nhs.uk, 2009), local radio and press are used.Steps have been taken to improve diet in schools, for example the much publicized Jamie Oliver campaign (Oliver, 2009), but school life is a relatively small part of a child's life; most life skills, including cooking, are learnt at home. Nonetheless, school involvement is welcomed, and school caterers are invited to participate in the course.

To counterbalance what might seem to adults like a return to school, other locality groups have been invited to take part, such as representatives from local luncheon clubs and dieticians. To facilitate inclusion of exercise in the course, the plan includes the contribution of physiotherapists and local Walking for Health (Ramblers, 2009) representatives. Multiagency meetings are essential to develop and implement this action plan. All stakeholders who are envisaged to participate will be invited, including representatives from local radio and TV and the Counterweight organization, with regard to a 'Buddy' maintenance programme to support patients to continue with improved lifestyle choices after the course.

It is planned to 'brainstorm' ideas, using local expertise to ensure that all avenues have been explored, and to develop a programme. This will help to identify any potential problems that need to be addressed. This will also allow us to check speaker availability and to ensure that each person is clear about session objectives. The authors intend to foster a team philosophy that is non-judgmental and demonstrates unconditional positive regard. Therefore, the first session will include healthy snacks and drinks, aiming to create a relaxed atmosphere to promote patient confidence and good discussion. *Table 12.3* highlights the proposed programme outline.

Following the success of a Healthy Lifestyle Fête at the practice, it is proposed that the people running local resources and services be invited to plan a 'Weigh Forward Fête' to showcase the course and the services that are available in the community. Local retailers will be asked whether they can award vouchers to patients receiving income support. PCT approval will be obtained to invite local multidisciplinary staff to run stalls that give information about their services. This 'free publicity' could make such showcasing worthwhile to all stakeholders. The fête provides the opportunity to market the course to families and sign them up to future courses. To ensure equity, we intend that subsequent courses will be offered to families who identify themselves, as well as to those families that we identify.

## Objective 4

Human, material and financial resources, and access, were also considered.

**Table 12.3 Weigh Forward weight management programme**

| | |
|---|---|
| **Week 1** | Introduction to the course<br>Discuss how confidentiality will be maintained<br>Discuss whether to weigh in front of other people<br>or in private<br>Introduce food diaries<br>Discuss and demonstrate BMI and how to calculate risk<br>using waist measurement calculations; anyone who wishes<br>can 'have a go' |
| **Week 2** | Presentation from a dietician who is a childhood<br>obesity specialist |
| **Week 3** | Presentation from the catering manager from local<br>schools—discussion on making healthy choices |
| **Week 4** | Presentation from a physiotherapist about the value of<br>walking, cycling etc, plus possibly demonstrating some<br>home-based exercises which group members can try<br>out with supervision (distribution of vouchers from local<br>bicycle retailer if available)<br>*OR*<br>Presentation from the local Walking Group. Possibly<br>plan a short walk in the area (depending on time of year).<br>Distribute pedometers which have been obtained free of<br>charge from a drug representative |
| **Week 5** | Presentation about healthy recipes (distribution<br>of healthy food vouchers from local supermarkets<br>if available) |
| **Week 6** | Round-up and evaluation<br>Presentation from a counterweight 'buddy' leading<br>to planning for a maintenance programme with<br>course members |

### Human resources

*Clients*

The authors agreed that the clients attending the service would bring a wealth
of experience to the group, which must be acknowledged and used.

## Course staff

Practice nurses are well placed to deliver health promotion initiatives; indeed, WIPP NHS (2009) state that practice nurses are central to the provision of information and support to enable patients to make appropriate choices for their health. In this way, the service should be acceptable. Meeting objective 1 ensured the approval of the practice manager, who agreed to include the healthcare assistants and administrative team in service development and delivery, as appropriate. It was agreed that practice nurses would induct new team members to the service, giving training as required, within existing protected learning time.

Meeting objective 3 indicated the use of a multiagency approach, therefore representatives of other locality groups are invited to take part and inducted at planning meetings.

## Time

In line with Government initiatives for widening access and increasing patient choice (DH, 2008b), the surgery has extended hours twice weekly until 8 pm. It was proposed that the course be held in these hours as they are also after work and school times. Babies and toddlers are welcome to avoid childcare problems.

## Venue

A large treatment room, which can accommodate 12 people within health and safety regulations, is used for the sessions. We hope to recruit 10–12 people (two to three families) per course.

## Stationery and marketing materials

Stationery is required to market the course. Participant invitations will involve administration time and cost of phone calls or postage. Posters will be developed at minimal cost using surgery IT and printing facilities.

## Session equipment

Scales are available at no cost. Venepuncture equipment is available; the cost of blood tests required would be acceptable, as they are for any patient, at any point of contact, if identified as necessary. Health promotion leaflets and posters are freely available. Laptop and projector are available for powerpoint or DVD presentations. Foodstuffs and vouchers might be available from local retailers.

## Objective costing

Costing is based on six-week courses, run eight times per year, and takes into account a variety of sundries plus human resources, as follows:

* Practice nurse
* Dietician/physiotherapist
* Walking for Health
* School meals
* Various foodstuffs.

### Potential cost benefits

It is difficult to predict actual savings accurately when planning a health promotion project (Ewles and Simnett, 2003). Indeed, when considering this service development there is no valid or reliable way of evaluating whether, as a direct result of this service alone, any person avoided developing disease, or improved their prognosis in the future—they may merely have not developed disease in the way that some people who smoke 40 cigarettes per day for 40 years develop smoking-related diseases. Furthermore, for some patients there are other confounding variables that could influence outcomes. For example, an overweight patient who is hypertensive could have his/her health potential improved by taking appropriate medication; and an overweight smoker could have his health potential improved through smoking cessation. Therefore, behaviour changes which occur concurrently can be assumed to have a cumulative effect on health potential, but it is difficult to extrapolate the exact benefit of each. However, reduction in risk will result in reduction in disease and in costs associated with appointments and prescriptions (Counterweight Project Team 2005a; 2005b).

Some examples of treatment costs for diabetes, one condition for which obesity is a major risk factor, are listed *Table 12.4*. All of these complications can affect one person. Diabetes UK (2009) estimate that 1 000 000 people are yet to be diagnosed. The UK Prospective Diabetes Study (UKPDS) proved, with research spanning 30 years, that good early control of glucose, blood pressure, BMI and cholesterol levels lead to better clinical outcomes (UKPDS Group, 1998; Diabetes UK, 2009). These are all adversely affected by obesity.

Arguably, the potential cost–benefits from this service are considerable, and the potential reduction in untimely mortality is of inestimable value. Targeting childhood obesity is a responsibility of all health practitioners and managers.

---

**Table 12.4 Treatment costs for diabetes**

**Typical treatment regimen:**
Metformin 500 mg, twice daily: £12 per annum
Add Glimepiride 1 mg: £37 per annum.
Add Pioglitazone 15 mg: approximately £300 per annum

**When triple therapy fails:**
Add insulin, e.g. Mixtard 5 x 3 ml: £960 per annum
Plus testing strips, lancets etc

Annual retinal screening

Complications of diabetes incur further costs, for example:
Glaucoma therapy
Leg ulcer treatment
Coronary Artery Bypass Graft—up to £20 000 in total

Costs sourced from Joint Formulary Committee (2009); and PbR National Tariff

---

## Objectives 5 and 6

Having stated that evaluation is unlikely to reveal actual cost savings or benefits, evaluation is paramount to the ongoing sustainability of this service. Patient satisfaction is important, therefore formative and summative evaluation is planned to show how the service is perceived by patients. The service will be monitored formatively through weekly notation of numbers attending and interest shown. Summative evaluation will be undertaken using questionnaires: one distributed at the beginning of the course, seeking patient's expectations; another distributed after course completion to measure whether patient expectations were met by the end of the programme.

Data will also be gathered to summatively evaluate levels of risk as per the literature. Actual weight-loss, percentage of body weight lost, BMI, waist measurements, and blood pressure will be recorded. If appropriate, blood tests, such as high-density lipoprotein, low-density lipoprotein, triglycerides and $HbA_{1c}$, will be audited as markers of improvement. The findings from evaluation will be fed back to patients in appropriate language to encourage continuation with behaviour change, and to market the service to patients who are considering take-up. In addition, the findings will be fed back to the practice team and the PCT. From the evaluation, the authors will negotiate an acceptable maintenance programme for course participants.

## Conclusion

This chapter has outlined the development of a weight management programme in rural Leicestershire. An adapted version of the Ewles and Simnett (2003) planning and evaluation cycle was used to guide and structure programme planning and this was supported by the development of SMART objectives. Planning gave detailed consideration to how each objective would be met. When planning a health promotion service, it is important that such attention is paid to detail. This increases the chance of success at both strategic and operational levels. In this instance, at strategic level, a substantive health needs analysis led to prioritization of need and the development of realistic aims and feasible objectives, which led to the development of a strategy that was accepted by the local PCT. Success at operational level is yet to be established when the service is rolled out. However, sound planning with attention to detail has given the authors the confidence that the service will be well received and successful.

*The Weigh Forward programme takes a broad approach that tackles the problem of obesity from a community perspective. The project uses a multiprofessional approach to identify effective strategies for health promotion that recognizes the importance of establishing healthy behaviours within families. Obesity has significant links to the development of certain long-term conditions and in the management of others. This project highlights the opportunities that nursing professionals have in making a difference to both current and future health.*

Centers for Disease Control and Prevention (2009) Health Consequences. www.cdc.gov/obesity/causes/health.html (accessed 16 November 2009)

Counterweight (2005a) The impact of obesity on drug prescribing in primary care. http://tinyurl.com/yhlsb6o (accessed 16 November 2009)

Counterweight (2005b) Obesity impacts on general practice appointments. http://tinyurl.com/y9sm4zq (accessed 16 November 2009)

DH (2005) *The General Medical Services Statements of Entitlements 2005 onwards.* DH, London. ref: 4567

DH (2007) Health risk and costs of obesity. http://tinyurl.com/ylq8wg4 (accessed 16 November 2009)

DH (2008a) Healthy Weight, Healthy Lives: A Cross-Government strategy for England. http://tinyurl.com/clbu4r (accessed 16 November 2009)

DH (2008b) *NHS Choices: delivering for the NHS*. DH, London. ref: 9432

DH (2009) Obesity. http://tinyurl.com/4952uj (accessed 16 November 2009)

Diabetes UK (2009) Benefits of early Type 2 diabetes control felt years later. http://tinyurl.com/yha99ge (accessed 16 November 2009)

Ewles L, Simnett I (2003) *Promoting Health: A Practical Guide*. 5th edn. Bailliere Tindall, London

Foresight (2007) Tacking Obesities: Future Choices—Project Report. www.foresight.gov.uk/Obesity/17.pdf (accessed 16 November 2009)

Haslam D, Sattar M, Lean M (2006) ABC of obesity. Obesity—time to wake up. *BMJ* **333**(7569): 640–2

MEND (2009) Fitter, healthier, happier families. www.mendprogramme.org (accessed 16 November 2009)

Must A, Spadano J, Coakley EH, Field AE, Colditz G, Dietz WH (1999) The disease burden associated with overweight and obesity. *JAMA* **282**(16): 1523–9

National Audit Office (2001) Tackling Obesity in England. http://tinyurl.com/yhz99vn (accessed 16 November 2009)

National Obesity Forum (2009a) Childhood Obesity. http://tinyurl.com/yfmv25w (accessed 16 November 2009)

National Obesity Forum (2009b) Long-term Effects. http://tinyurl.com/yz63qqs (accessed 16 November 2009)

National Prescribing Centre (2009) Obesity. http://tinyurl.com/yklq4r9 (accessed 16 November 2009)

NHS Information Centre (2008) The National Child Measurement Programme results. www.ncmp.ic.nhs.uk (accessed 16 November 2009)

NHS Modernisation Agency (2004) Ten steps to SMART objectives. http://tinyurl.com/37xky9 (accessed 14 December 2009)

nhs.uk (2009) change4life. www.nhs.uk/Change4Life (accessed 16 November 2009)

Oliver J (2009) School Dinners. www.jamieoliver.com/school-dinners (accessed 16 November 2009)

Ramblers (2009) Walking for health. http://tinyurl.com/ylerp5f (accessed 16 November 2009)

SIGN (2003) Management of obesity in children and young people. www.sign.ac.uk/pdf/sign69.pdf (accessed 16 November 2009)

UKPDS Group (1998) Intensive blood-glucose control with sulphonylureas or insulin compared with conventional treatment and risk of complications in patients with type 2 diabetes (UKPDS 33). *Lancet* **352**(9131): 837–53

Weight-control Information Network (2007) Do you know the health risks of being overweight? http://tinyurl.com/yl5drfq (accessed 16 November 2009)

WIPP NHS (2009) Role of the general practice nurse in contributing to key functions of the primary care trust. http://tinyurl.com/yefqr3s (accessed 15 December 2009)

Zaninotto P, Wardle H, Stamatakis E, Mindell J, Head J (2006) Forecasting Obesity to 2010. http://tinyurl.com/yjzfqys (accessed 16 November 2009)

# CHAPTER 13

# Problem alcohol use

*Ira Unell*

Alcohol has been accessible to almost every society, culture and tribe for centuries. Some religions, such as Islam and some evangelical Christian groups, have rejected the use of alcohol, but they are a minority. Despite these exceptions, it is the most popular drug in the world. Most people will drink relatively small quantities of alcohol for the whole of their lives and suffer no adverse consequences. A significant minority will drink heavily for a period of time, increasing the risk of health or social problems, but manage to avoid lasting damage. As we grow older, most (by no means all) of us will reduce our alcohol consumption as we gain more responsibilities, have families, and acquire cars and mortgages. This chapter will cover the consequences of heavy drinking over time. Many people will use alcohol problematically, if only for a short time, and come to a degree of harm as a result. This chapter will enable you to:

- Assess a patient's drinking
- Understand the health, familial, and social consequences
  of problematic drinking
- Understand the treatment options
- Consider how you might help to minimize harm from
  problematic drinking.

## Background

Alcohol is not only the most popular drug in the UK, but also in the world. The per capita consumption of alcohol has been steadily climbing in the UK while falling in most other European countries. In 1963, per capita alcohol consumption was approximately four times higher in France than the UK. By 2003, the UK had surpassed French consumption (9.6 litres of pure alcohol per capita compared with 9.3) (Institute of Alcohol Studies [IAS], 2008a). In England, in 2006, 72% of men and 57% of women had alcohol on at least one day in the week before being asked/consulted (NHS Information Centre, 2008). A smaller proportion—12% of men and 7% of women—had a drink every day in the previous week. Most people who drink moderate amounts of alcohol have no or minimal risk of problems associated with alcohol use. Those who drink more than the recommended limits increase the risk of disease and adverse social consequences. For those who drink only a little more than the recommended limits, the additional risks are marginal. However, the more you drink, the more your risk of disease and adverse social consequences increases. Those who drink at much higher levels have much higher risk.

The pattern of drinking is also important, as well as the amount that people consume every week. Heavy drinking in a short time increases the risk of accident or violence, crime associated with drinking, contracting a sexually transmitted disease, or unplanned pregnancy. Withdrawal symptoms from drinking are usually unpleasant, but if associated with chronic or very heavy drinking, can be dangerous or even life-threatening.

## Addiction

Addiction is a difficult word to define. However defined, it includes the idea that after repeated use of a drug, an individual may feel a compulsion to continue taking it. The word is usually (not always) associated with the notion that addiction is harmful to the individual, his/her family, and society as a whole. Sometimes the harm is minimal and other times deadly.

Addiction usually means that the individual is psychologically dependent (i.e. experiences discomfort such as anxiety, low mood, craving for the drug) and/or physically dependent (i.e. characteristic, unpleasant and sometimes dangerous withdrawal symptoms appear, at least for a time, when the drug is no longer used). Addiction is associated with drug tolerance (feeling the need for increased dosage of the drug to achieve the same effect). Some people feel that the word 'addiction' is judgmental and disparaging, in that it implies that the 'addict' is no longer able to control his/her behaviour. Often the term 'drug/alcohol misuse' or 'problem alcohol/drug use' is used instead.

People with alcohol problems usually have a variety of other problems associated with their drinking. It is essential to negotiate with the patient about his/her needs and what should take priority. While it is true that reducing or stopping drinking will almost always help any or all of the problems, this must be managed with care. For instance, sudden abstinence or dramatic reduction of drinking for heavy drinkers can bring on dangerous withdrawal symptoms, from nausea and vomiting to hallucinations and seizures. This should always be done with the advice of a doctor, nurse, or alcohol treatment agency. It could be the case that other associated problems need to be addressed before the drinking (e.g. homelessness).

There are many words which can be used to describe an alcohol problem, such as dependence, addiction, or alcoholism. In this chapter, the term 'problem alcohol use' will be used. The terms 'addict' and 'alcoholism' are often applied to those who find it very difficult to stop drinking and have suffered severe consequences, including dangerous withdrawal symptoms. Other publications or groups who may use words like dependence or alcoholic will be referred to. These terms imply that the individual may be suffering from a disease which has a characteristic set of signs, symptoms, and natural history, and that he/she can no longer control his/her drinking. This point of view is often referred to as the disease concept of chemical dependency or alcoholism.

## Assessing alcohol problems

Most alcohol treatment agencies will have their own system of assessing alcohol problems. Doctors often use DSM-III or IV (Diagnostic and Statistical Manual of Mental Disorders) or ICD-10 (International Classification of Disease) criteria for alcohol dependence, misuse or harmful use. The heaviest drinking can lead to dependence.

### Defining alcohol dependence

One way of defining alcohol dependence is provided by one of the standard systems of diagnosis used by psychiatrists, *The ICD-10 Classification of Mental and Behavioural Disorders: Clinical Descriptions and Diagnostic Guidelines*, Criteria for the Alcohol Dependence Syndrome (World Health Organization [WHO], 2004). According to these criteria, for a diagnosis of alcohol dependence to be present, three or more of the following signs should have occurred together for at least one month or, if persisting for periods of less than one month, should have occurred together repeatedly within a 12-month period:

- A strong desire or sense of compulsion to consume alcohol
- Impaired capacity to control drinking in terms of its onset, termination, or levels of use, as evidenced by alcohol being often taken in larger amounts or over a longer period than intended; or by a persistent desire to or unsuccessful efforts to reduce or control alcohol use
- A physiological withdrawal state when alcohol is reduced or ceased, as evidenced by the characteristic withdrawal syndrome for alcohol, or by use of the same (or closely related) substance with the intention of relieving or avoiding withdrawal symptoms

- Evidence of tolerance to the effects of alcohol, such that there is a need for significantly increased amounts of alcohol to achieve intoxication or the desired effect, or a markedly diminished effect with continued use of the same amount of alcohol
- Preoccupation with alcohol, as manifested by important alternative pleasures or interests being given up or reduced because of drinking; or a great deal of time being spent in activities necessary to obtain, take, or recover from the effects of alcohol
- Persistent alcohol use despite clear evidence of harmful consequences, as evidenced by continued use when the individual is actually aware, or may be expected to be aware, of the nature and extent of harm.

## Calculating units of alcohol and calculating consumption

Alcohol consumption is measured in units; one unit is 10 ml or 8 grams of pure alcohol. This is found in half a pint of 3.5% beer, lager or cider, a pub measure of spirit, or a small (125 ml) glass of 9% wine. Note that many beers, ciders and lager are much stronger today at 4–5% and up to 9%, and the wine we drink today is often 12–14%. In most pubs and restaurants, the 125 ml glass has been replaced by the 175 ml glass, or a supersize 250 ml. Some pubs have increased their measure of spirits from 25 ml to 35 ml (Elliot and Ford, 2008). In calculating units of alcohol, take into account the strength of the alcohol that people drink. Many of the heaviest drinkers will simply not be able to remember how much they have had. 'Street drinkers' often drink with other street drinkers and pass around the beer, cider or wine, so may not be able to accurately estimate their consumption. Other ways of assessing consumption can also be made by finding out how many days and how many hours each day people spend drinking. Also, the careful recording of withdrawal symptoms and physical and mental health can help an assessment.

### Safe limits

The Department of Health (DH) (2005) suggests that men should not drink more than three to four units of alcohol per day and women not more than two or three units of alcohol per day. After heavy drinking, a break of 28 hours is recommended. Pregnant women or women trying to conceive should not drink alcohol and if they do choose to drink, they should limit their drinking to one or two units once or twice a week (National Institute for Health and Clinical Excellence [NICE], 2008). During the first three months of pregnancy, the foetus is most at risk from the adverse effects of alcohol (NHS Choices, 2008). Regular alcohol consumption in excess of the recommended daily guideline can be a contributory factor in a number of long-term health conditions.

---

**Reflection**

- You might try working out your own or a colleagues' weekly alcohol consumption
- Think about the people you have nursed. Do you routinely assess a patient's alcohol consumption?

---

### Liver function tests

Liver function tests (LFTs) are usually a good indicator of current and, to some extent, previous drinking habits. There are many types of LFT used diagnostically for a variety of conditions. The two most relevant for heavy drinking are gamma glutamyltransferase (GGT) and bilirubin. GGT usually ranges between 11–50 iu/l for men, and 7–32 iu/l for women.

GGT is involved in glutathione metabolism, which plays an important role in antioxidant defence, and moving other amino acids across the cell membrane. GGT can be raised because of a range of problems such as myocardial infarction, diabetes, obesity, pancreatic disease and smoking, as well as heavy drinking. Some drugs such as barbiturates and phenytoin can also cause elevated GGT. Having noted the exceptions, raised GGT are a good indicator of excessive drinking. For those with a long history of alcohol problems, raised GGT can be in the hundreds, or well over a thousand.

Bilirubin has a normal range of up to 17 umol/l of blood. Bilirubin comes from the breakdown of haemoglobin and can be elevated by other problems than those related to heavy drinking, such as viral hepatitis, blocked bile ducts or cirrhosis. When bilirubin accumulates, it is apparent as jaundice. Different laboratories may have somewhat different ranges for both GGT and bilirubin (British Liver Trust, 2008).

## Health consequences of heavy drinking

### Withdrawal symptoms

Withdrawal symptoms from alcohol may be mild and short-lived, such as a hangover, which could include nausea, vomiting, headache, fatigue, anxiety, tremor, and sweating. Major withdrawal symptoms from heavy problematic drinking can include hallucinations (usually auditory or visual), seizures, disorientation and confusion, tachycardia, hypertension and hyperventilation. Major withdrawals should be treated with tranquilizers such as chlordiazepoxide, in a decreasing regimen over a period of two weeks (Joint Formulary Committee, 2009). This will prevent the dangerous or life-threatening symptoms such as seizures or hallucinations.

Women may be especially vulnerable to the consequences of heavy drinking, as the same quantity of alcohol will have a larger effect because of differences in body fat and size compared with men. Women who are pregnant, particularly during the first trimester, should abstain from alcohol and if they do drink, it should be no more than one or two units once or twice a week (NICE, 2008).

---

**Reflection**

- Look at *Table 13.1*
- Consider the medical problems related to excessive drinking
- Which of these may be related to the development of a long-term condition?
- Consider the consequences of excessive drinking in patients with existing long-term conditions.

---

## Alcohol as a cause of death

Excessive alcohol consumption is directly linked to the development of cirrhosis of the liver (*Table 13.2*). In 2005, 4160 people in England and Wales died from alcoholic liver disease, and mortality data shows a worrying increase in deaths from cirrhosis in the 25–34 year age groups (DH, 2007). Heavy drinking is a contributory factor in the development of cardiovascular disease, hypertension and stroke. Data suggest that the magnitude of increased risk for developing hypertension in men and women is four- and three-fold respectively (DH, 2007). In addition, men have a 1.7-fold increased risk of developing coronary heart disease compared with a 1.3-fold increased risk for women (DH, 2007).

## Alcohol and mental health

Alcohol can be a significant cause of mental health problems, and those who already have a mental health problem are at high risk of developing an alcohol problem. In practice it is often difficult to tell which came first; the mental health problem or alcohol problem. The best results seem to come from treating them simultaneously. When the two problems come together, it is often

## Table 13.1 Medical problems related to alcohol

**Nervous system**
Acute intoxication blackouts
Persistent brain damage: Wernicke's encephalopathy and
Korsakoff's psychosis
Cerebellar degeneration
Dementia
Cerebrovascular disease: stroke, especially in young people
Subarachnoid haemorrhage
Subdural haematoma after head injury
Withdrawal symptoms: tremor, hallucinations, fits
Nerve and muscle damage: weakness, paralysis, burning sensation
in hands and feet

**Liver**
Infiltration of liver with fat
Alcoholic hepatitis
Cirrhosis and eventual liver failure
Liver cancer

**Gastrointestinal system**
Reflux of acid into the oesophagus
Tearing and occasionally rupture of the oesophagus
Cancer of the oesophagus
Gastritis
Aggravation and impaired healing of peptic ulcers
Diarrhoea and impaired absorption of food
Chronic inflammation of the pancreas leading (in some cases) to
diabetes and malabsorption of food

**Nutrition**
Malnutrition from reduced intake of food, toxic effects of alcohol on
intestine, and impaired metabolism, leading to weight-loss
Obesity, particularly in the early stages of heavy drinking

**Heart and circulatory system**
Abnormal rhythms
High blood pressure
Chronic heart muscle damage leading to heart failure

**Respiratory system**
Pneumonia from inhalation of vomit
Overproduction of cortisol leading to obesity, acne, increased facial hair,
and high blood pressure
Condition mimicking over-activity of the thyroid with loss of weight,

anxiety, palpitations, sweating, and tremor

Severe fall in blood sugar, sometimes leading to coma

Intense facial flushing in many diabetics taking the anti-diabetic drug chlorpropamide

**Reproductive system**

In men, loss of libido, reduced potency, shrinkage in size of testes and penis, reduced or absent sperm formation and so infertility, and loss of sexual hair

In women, sexual difficulties, menstrual irregularities, and shrinkage of breasts and external genitalia

**Occupation and accidents**

Impaired work performance and decision-making

Increased risk and severity of accidents

**The foetus, the child and the family**

Damage to the foetus and foetal alcohol syndrome

Acute intoxication in young children produces hypothermia, low blood sugar levels, depressed respiration

Effect on physical development and behaviour of child through heavy drinking by parents

Interaction of alcohol with medicinal substances

Increased likelihood of unwanted effects of drugs

Reduced effectiveness of medicines

From: Institute of Alcohol Studies (2008b)

---

**Table 13.2 Estimates of proportion of deaths attributable to alcohol from a variety of conditions**

| Condition % | Attributable to alcohol |
|---|---|
| Cancer of oesophagus | 14–75% |
| Cancer of liver | 15–29% |
| Cancer of female breast | 3–4% |
| Hypertension | 5–11% |
| Chronic pancreatitis | 60–84% |
| Acute pancreatitis | 24–42% |
| Falls | 23–35% |
| Drownings | 30–38% |
| Fire injuries | 38–45% |
| Suicide | 27–41% |
| Assault | 27–47% |

From: Institute of Alcohol Studies (2008b)

referred to as 'dual diagnosis'. In many areas there is still a gap between the alcohol treatment services and the mental health services where coordinated treatment is called for, but the means and will to provide it is lacking.

Many people with alcohol problems will tell you that they are depressed. Often the source of their depression comes from the problems associated with heavy drinking and also the effect that alcohol can have on the brain. The reduction of consumption or abstinence is often enough to resolve the feelings of depression, but there will always be some problem drinkers who have more persistent and severe depression requiring treatment. Depressive symptoms are difficult to treat psychologically while someone is drinking heavily, and antidepressant drugs are less effective for those who drink any more than moderate amounts of alcohol. Note that patients who attempt suicide, for whatever reason, often drink heavily before an attempt.

Those suffering from schizophrenia or other psychotic disorders also frequently develop a drink problem, especially when they first develop symptoms. Later, they may drink in response to their symptoms. Alcohol can temporarily help with psychotic symptoms for some people, but withdrawals usually make symptoms worse. Those diagnosed with a personality disorder are even more likely to simultaneously have a drink problem. In addition, it is common for people to experience agoraphobia during alcohol withdrawal. It will usually fade away if the drinking levels improve, but sometimes the symptoms can persist and require intervention, usually behavioural or cognitive/behavioural therapy (IAS, 2007a)

For persistent, heavy drinkers, alcoholic amnesia can be a problem. The heaviest drinkers can develop Wernicke's encepalopathy, which can turn into a more permanent condition called Korsakoff's psychosis. This is caused by a deficiency of thiamine, which comes from poor eating habits and the malabsorption of thiamine in the presence of alcohol. The symptoms are very similar in some ways to dementia suffered by older people:

- Visual problems such as double vision, abnormal eye movements or drooping eyelids
- Poor muscle coordination or uncoordinated walking
- Memory problems, particularly short-term
- Hallucinations.

## Alcohol and other drugs

Alcohol alters the effect of both illegal and prescribed drugs. For example, using alcohol with benzodiazepines will enhance the effect of the alcohol, so the person who takes both might seem to be very intoxicated, but will only have consumed a small quantity of alcohol.

Alcohol will increase the risk of overdose for those who use heroin or other opiates such as methadone. Also, it will make drugs prescribed for schizophrenia, depression and other mental health problems less effective.

# Social problems

Excessive drinking is associated with a large proportion of crime. Research suggests that 63% of sentenced prisoners and 39% of women prisoners admit to hazardous drinking before imprisonment. Alcohol-related crime is estimated to cost the UK £7.3 billion per year (Alcohol Concern, 2008). Both the perpetrators of violence and victims of violence have often been drinking heavily before the offence, including 60–70% of all homicides (IAS, 2007b). In addition, there are the deaths and injuries which arise directly from drinking, such as drink–driving. In 2001, there were 78 684 convictions for driving under the influence of alcohol in England. In addition, there were an estimated 540 deaths caused by driving under the influence, plus another 13 840 injuries in 2006 (IAS, 2007c). Add to this the cost in unemployment, benefits, insurance, police, health costs, court and prison costs, and it is easy to see why the total cost of alcohol use to society is huge—estimated at approximately £20 billion in 2006 for England and Wales. To offset this cost, the Inland Revenue collects approximately £13.26 billion in tax (IAS, 2007d).

## *Family consequences*

Having one or more members of the family with a drink problem can have a profound detrimental effect on the other members of the family. Problem alcohol use is frequently associated with domestic violence and marital disharmony. Financial and employment problems can occur, adding to the discord. Often sexual relations suffer as well. Children brought up in a home with a problem drinking parent(s) are at risk of developing a number of problems, such as:

- A greater likelihood of early drinking and/or problem drinking later in life
- Behavioural problems
- Inconsistent parenting
- School problems and underachievement
- Attachment problems
- Child abuse or neglect.

The risks listed are not inevitable, and much can be done to limit the damage. There is good evidence that the following family characteristics reduce the harm suffered by children from their parent's problematic drinking:

- One stable parent, grandparent, family member or adult
- Maintenance of family rituals (e.g. birthdays)
- Absence of domestic violence, minimum aggression in family
- Consistent parenting
- Good communication between family members
- Parent(s) in treatment for their alcohol problem.

# Living with and helping long-term problem drinkers

It has often been said that an 'addiction' is a relapsing condition. Many people, over their lifetime, will develop one or more problems associated with drinking. The large majority will not come for help and many of those will reduce their drinking with no professional help. Most observers agree that as we become older, we drink less anyway. This is not always the case, however. Retirement, bereavement, unemployment and other life transitions can lead to problematic drinking at any age.

## The course of problem drinking

People who develop a drug or alcohol problem often do not recognize the problems which are being caused (pre-contemplation), but eventually start to think about the consequences and weigh them against the benefits of continued use (contemplation). Eventually, they may decide to think about changing their behaviour (preparation), start to change their behaviour (action), maintain that change for some time (maintenance), and either maintain the change for long enough to move out of the cycle or relapse. Once they relapse for a long enough time, they often go back to either the pre-contemplation or contemplation stage. Some people never move from pre-contemplation to contemplation, and others never move beyond contemplation. That is, they realize that they have a problem with the drug, but the problems in changing and benefits from continuing outweigh the perceived benefits of reducing or becoming abstinent (*Figure 13.1*). Prochaska and DiClemente (1994) have proposed a scheme called 'the cycle of change' for understanding the relapsing nature of 'addiction'.

## Helping problem drinkers to change

The best way to help is to determine where the problem drinker may be on the cycle of change. If, for instance, they are in the 'pre-contemplation' stage, you could help by getting them to think about the advantages and disadvantages of their current drinking. (If they see no benefit in continuing

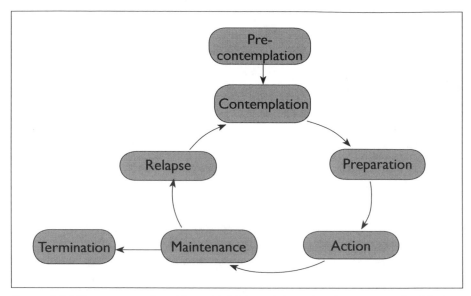

*Figure 13.1 The course of problem drinking and the relapsing nature of addiction*

they may be ready to think about cutting down or stopping.) It is better if they can tell you the benefits and problems associated with their drinking, rather then you telling them. Evidence shows that they are more likely to move to the next stage—think about how to change, if they accept that it is their decision rather than someone else's (IAS, 2001).

If, and only if, they have decided that they want to make a change, you can help them to decide how to do it. It might involve finding help from a non-statutory alcohol advice centre, GP, NHS alcohol treatment team, or a self-help group such as Alcoholics Anonymous (AA). Remember that if significant withdrawal symptoms are likely, or the problem drinker has other physical or mental health problems, then the help of an experienced nurse or doctor will be necessary. They may want to prescribe tranquilizers to prevent some of the more dangerous symptoms.

Helping problem drinkers to slowly reduce their consumption is usually a good idea. Sudden abstinence is often more difficult and, as stated previously, can be dangerous in some circumstances. Small but steady reduction to a safer level is a good start. Once a safer level of abstinence has been achieved, you can help by talking to the problem drinker about how he/she might avoid a relapse. This could involve trying to reduce some of the 'cues' for drinking heavily, such as finding someone to talk to if they feel low in mood, avoiding heavy drinking friends, or exercise. Finding other ways of spending time and money is usually helpful and lots of support from family and friends is always beneficial. One or more days a week of total abstinence can help get people out of the habit of relying on a drink.

Relapse or 'lapse' from a programme of controlled drinking or abstinence is common. It need not be the end of the world. The sooner it ends and the less damage it causes, the better. Remind the problem drinker of the progress he/she has made and help him/her to learn from mistakes and how they can be avoided the next time.

## Abstinence or controlled drinking?

There is a long-standing and continuing debate about the possibility of controlled drinking, that is, planned reduction to safer limits of drinking, or complete abstinence. Some people, particularly those who advocate a 'discase model' of drinking say that an 'alcoholic' cannot control his/her drinking even with help, and therefore total abstinence is the only practical method (IAS, 2001). Others say that there is evidence that many people can 'unlearn' their previous drinking habit and relearn a less harmful pattern of drinking. It might be the case that the most long-standing and damaged problem drinkers are the least likely to follow a planned reduced drinking habit, but this is by no means always the case. Also, there is no convincing evidence that planned abstinence is any more likely to prevent relapse than controlled drinking.

---

### Reflection

- Have you met any patients who have been problem drinkers?
- Consider what steps you might realistically take to help them
- Identify agencies and sources in your local area that might be available to help you.

---

# Treatment

## Community treatment

Treatment for alcohol problems includes a number of activities and is available from a variety of agencies. Alcohol advice centres or alcohol counselling agencies, usually within the voluntary sector, offer assessment and a number of treatment options, such as supportive counselling, motivational interviewing and brief interventions. The Probation Service often has a team for helping offenders with their drink problems. Also, the NHS will usually (although not always) have a specialist alcohol treatment team with a community base. This is often the team that deals with people with the most difficult problems associated with drinking, as well as pregnant women with drinking problems and those who simultaneously have an alcohol and mental health problem (dual diagnosis). If necessary, they can arrange for a hospital bed for detoxification. Most GPs and primary care teams offer some help or at least advice and referral to another agency.

Although there is a wide variety of support available, community based treatments for alcohol problems do not necessarily offer a clear pathway of care to individuals seeking help and support. The DH has recognized that agencies need to work together need to assess need and provide coordinated services for problem drinkers (DH, 2005). While a care pathway may be useful, it is important to remember that interventions may need to be considered using a more individualized approach.

## Residential treatment

For those who need continuing support, there are 'dry houses' and therapeutic communities which offer a 24-hour residential programme. They usually ask people to stay for between six and 12 months, or sometimes longer, and some offer rehousing or supported housing after the residential programme has been completed. They are most often abstinence-only, and drinking can lead to eviction. They are expensive, and while the local authority may be prepared to pay the cost, they will need to be convinced that community treatment has been tried and failed.

## Self-help groups

In addition there are self-help groups such as AA. AA has been imported from the US and is entirely voluntary. It receives no government and rarely any charitable funding through choice, since it values its independence. Most areas have AA meetings which anyone can attend, sometimes on every day of the week. An additional benefit is that it supplies a ready-made group of friends who often plan social activities together. It is for 'alcoholics' only, but there are sometimes separate groups for family support or aimed at young drinkers. AA sees 'alcoholism' as a disease and says that the best test to determine whether or not you suffer from it is the amount of damage caused to your health, family, and society at large as a result of drinking, and the inability to stop drinking once you have started. According to this perspective, total abstinence is the only alternative to continued destructive drinking once it is clear that you are an 'alcoholic'. AA has proved to be an enormous help for some, but others find the AA-style of group meetings and the exposing of personal problems to a group of strangers off-putting.

# Conclusion

This chapter has explored problematic alcohol use. Demographic evidence has highlighted that alcohol misuse and problematic drinking is increasing and as a result is a significant health issue. The links between alcohol and the development of and the prognosis of many long-term conditions has been clearly highlighted. The consequences of alcohol misuse impact not only on the individuals' physiological and psychological health, but also have social, environmental and community implications. Health professionals have an important role to play in identifying problem drinkers, providing support and advice to enable them to modify or change their lifestyle. Of equal importance is an understanding of the range of treatment and management options that are available so that they can direct and refer individuals and their families to other professionals and agencies.

Alcohol Concern (2008) *Alcohol and Crime*. Alcohol Concern, London

British Liver Trust (2008) *Alcohol and Crime*. British Liver Trust, Ringwood

DH (2005) *Alcohol Misuse Interventions: Guidance on developing a local programme of improvements*. DH, London. ref: 5694

DH (2007) *Safe. Sensible. Social. The next steps in the National Alcohol Strategy*. DH, London. ref: 8079

Elliot F, Ford R (2008) Pubs may be forced to offer smaller glass sizes for wine and spirits. http://tinyurl.com/6go2bn (accessed 12 November 2009)

IAS (2001) Alcohol Problems Causes and Prevention. http://tinyurl.com/yck999k (accessed 14 December 2009)

IAS (2007a) Alcohol and Mental Health. http://tinyurl.com/68hl9d (accessed 12 November 2009)

IAS (2007b) Alcohol and Crime. http://tinyurl.com/3bvfuc (accessed 12 November 2009)

IAS (2007c) Drinking and Driving. http://tinyurl.com/ykh3vft (accessed 12 November 2009)

IAS (2007d) Economic costs and benefits. http://tinyurl.com/yac35ba (accessed 12 November 2009)

IAS (2008a) *Alcohol and Harm in the UK and the EU*. IAS, London

IAS (2008b) Alcohol and Health. http://tinyurl.com/yb9wqfm (accessed 12 November 2009)

Joint Formulary Committee (2009) *British National Formulary* 58. September. BMJ Publishing Group Ltd and RPS Publishing, London

NHS Choices (2008) Know your limits. www.nhs.uk/units (accessed 12 November 2009)

NHS Information Centre (2008) Statistics on Alcohol: England, 2008. http://tinyurl.com/

y9lw6hu (accessed 12 November 2009)

NICE (2008) Antenatal care: full guidance. http://guidance.nice.org.uk/CG62/Guidance/pdf/ English (accessed 14 December 2009)

Prochaska JO, DiClemente CC (1994) *The Transtheoretical Approach: crossing traditional boundaries of therapy.* Krieger Publishing Company, New York

WHO (2004) The ICD-10 Classification of Mental and Behavioural Disorders: Clinical descriptions and diagnostic guidelines. http://tinyurl.com/ybtrnwn (accessed 14 December 2009)

## Further reading

Cleaver H, Unell I, Aldgate J (1999) *Children's Needs, Parenting Capacity: The Impact of parental mental illness, problem alcohol and drug use, and domestic violence on children's development.* The Stationery Office, London

Kroll B, Taylor A (2003) *Parental Substance Misuse and Child Welfare.* Jessica Kingsley Publishers, London

# CHAPTER 14

# Palliative care

*Debbie Lewis*

This chapter explores the concept of palliative care with regard to long-term conditions. It will help you to define palliative care, understand its historical perspective, and relate its key principles to the care of patients. Throughout the chapter, Government initiatives designed to enhance and standardize palliative care will be discussed, and their principles applied to the physical, psychological and social care of patients with long-term conditions in the palliative phase of their disease.

Reading this chapter and reflecting on your own experiences should enable you to achieve the following learning outcomes:

* To identify the goals of palliative care
* To identify the key service providers in meeting palliative care needs
* To explore how services are organized
* To recognize the role of informal care-givers.

## Background

Historically, palliative care evolved from the work of early religious organizations caring for the sick and destitute before concentrating its efforts on the relief of suffering of patients with a malignant disease. In the 21$^{st}$ century, it is acknowledged that the majority of deaths, rather than being caused by cancer, follow a period of chronic illness, such as heart disease, stroke, chronic respiratory disease, neurological disease, or dementia (Department of Health [DH], 2008). Recognition of this change in focus was heralded by the World Health Organization (WHO) in 2002, when it rewrote its frequently quoted definition of palliative care to encompass the wide range of patients who needed help and advice during the palliative care phase of their illness:

> *'Palliative care is an approach that improves the quality of life of patients and their families facing the problem associated with life-threatening illness, through the prevention and relief of suffering by means of early*

> *identification and impeccable assessment and treatment of pain and other problems, physical, psychosocial and spiritual'*
>
> World Health Organization (2009)

Expanding the remit of palliative care to include patients with long-term conditions brings with it a range of new issues and problems. The potential number of patients increases dramatically, with a corresponding increase in the potential workload for the health service. In the UK, 2800 per 1 000 000 die from cancer each year, of which it is estimated that 25–65% will need specialist palliative care support (Higginson, 1997). Compare this with the number of patients dying from other causes—6900 per 1 000 000—and we can see a huge increase in workload in the 21st century (Murtagh et al, 2004). This chapter will explore the capacity of existing services to meet this demand and discuss the adaption of the key principles of palliative care to meet the challenge of caring for patients with long-term illnesses.

## What is palliative care?

Palliative care is the active holistic care of patients and their families when a patient's disease is no longer responsive to curative treatment. The word 'palliative' derives from the Latin word *pallium*, meaning a cloak. Palliation therefore means to cloak over difficulties in order to reduce or eliminate unpleasant effects (Billings, 2007). The origins of palliative care stem back to the Middle Ages, when care and comfort was delivered by religious institutions to weary Christians journeying pilgrim routes (Saunders, 2005). In practice, the care administered was not limited to those travellers of the Christian faith, but encompassed the orphaned, sick and destitute. These early Christian refuges developed into the hospitals we are familiar with today. The word 'hospice' derived from the Latin word *horpes*, which originally meant a 'stranger' and evolved into *hospitalis* meaning 'friendly to a stranger' (Saunders, 2005).

The creation of St Christopher's Hospice in London by Cicely Saunders in 1967 (Clarke, 2004) recognized palliative care as a modern healthcare specialty. The focus of palliative care in its early days related almost exclusively to the care of patients with cancer (Payne et al, 2008), with efforts concentrated on relieving distressing physical symptoms in the last few weeks of a patient's life. Medical and nursing care delivered at this late stage of a patient's illness was called 'terminal care'. Today the terminology 'end-of-life care' is more commonly used with psychological, social and spiritual support seen as equally important as symptom relief (Saunders, 2005). The scope of palliative care widened in 1995 with the publication of the Calman–Hine Report (DH, 1995). This report called for palliative care services to increase their accessibility, enabling patients to obtain advice and support at any stage of their illness as opposed to simply gaining access at the end of life. This helped to ensure that patients could obtain advice when appropriate from palliative care specialists, optimizing their opportunity to have a high quality of life despite a potentially limited lifespan.

---

### Reflection

- Think about your recent clinical placement
- Did you look after a dying patient?
- Can you identify what condition or disease he/she was suffering from?

---

## Palliative care and long-term conditions

Palliative care services initially cared for patients with cancer and progressively degenerative diseases, such as motor neurone disease (Doyle et al, 2005). In an increasingly ageing population, the main causes of mortality are heart disease, cerebral vascular disorders, chronic respiratory disease, neurological disease and dementia (DH, 2008). It is now acknowledged that patients dying from such diseases face equally demanding physical, psychological and social challenges as those experienced by cancer patients. In fact, the daily long-term challenges of chronic conditions may be more stressful and cause a greater level of psychological and social dysfunction than the relatively predictable decline in function experienced by cancer patients (Ellenwood and Jenkins, 2007).

With regard to offering an equal service to these patients, the UK falls behind the USA, with only 5% of all patients referred to specialist palliative services having a diagnosis of non-malignant disease (Payne et al, 2008). In the USA, in a similar time frame, nearly 20% of patients referred suffered from a non-malignant disease (Fallon, 2005). Such discrepancies are influenced in part by the funding differences between the two countries. In America, Medicare provides funding to meet the needs of individual patients, while in the UK funding is given to palliative care services. This funding is inadequate with service providers relying heavily on monies from charities such as Macmillan Cancer Relief, Marie Curie Cancer Care, and the Sue Ryder Foundation Homes. Despite this difficulty, anecdotal evidence suggests that increasing numbers of patients with non-malignant disease are now being referred to hospital-based palliative care services and that staff are becoming more skilled in their care (Knight, 2006). Collating satisfactory statistics in an ageing population, however, is difficult. In the very elderly, the cause of death may be multifactorial or poorly defined (Driver et al, 2008).

In addition to funding difficulties, the judging of the patient's likely prognosis (known as prognostication) is considerably more difficult to assess in long-term conditions than in patients with cancer. In contrast to malignancy, where death generally follows a predicable decline in function, patients with long-term conditions suffer intermittent serious episodes of illness with gradually diminishing functional ability. In addition, active medical treatment may continue until the patient dies (Addington-Hall, 2008), reducing the window of opportunity for referral to palliative care services. Sudden death is also more common, particularly in patients with heart disease (Addington-Hall, 2008). Innovative models of care are suggested to counteract these problems with one-off consultations and short-term periods of intervention, as well as shared care (e.g. working alongside the patient's usual care providers) (Addington-Hall, 2008). The need to educate palliative care professionals about non-malignant conditions, as well as attracting specialists from other fields to palliative care, is also recognized (Addington-Hall, 2008).

## The goals of palliative care

The goals of palliative care were refined by the WHO in 2002 (*Table 14.1*). This work developed the earlier WHO statements of 2000, which related the principles of palliative care solely to patients with cancer. It is now recognized that the principles of palliative care apply to all patients with advanced life-threatening illness regardless of the cause.

## The organization of palliative care

Hospices are the institutions most commonly associated with the delivery of palliative care, but the majority of patients with long-term conditions will receive care from their normal healthcare providers (Payne et al, 2008). These providers may be hospital or care home staff, or the patient's local primary healthcare team. A primary healthcare team will typically consist of a GP, community nurses and social care support workers, delivering care within the patient's own home. The skills of such a team may be supplemented by the expertise of other professionals, including a community matron. This is a senior nurse with disease-specific or palliative care experience, fulfilling a role that evolved from the *NHS Improvement Plan* (DH, 2004). There are increasing numbers of such specialist nurses working with patients suffering from heart and respiratory diseases. The role aims to reduce the level of

---

**Table 14.1 Defining the goals of palliative care**

---

- Provides relief from pain and other distressing symptoms
- Affirms life and regards dying as a normal process
- Intends neither to hasten nor to postpone death
- Integrates the psychological and spiritual aspects of patients
- Offers a support system to help patients live as actively as possible until death
- Offers a support system to help the family cope during the patient's illness and in their bereavement
- Uses a team approach to address the needs of patients and their families, including bereavement counselling, if indicated
- Will enhance quality of life, and may also positively influence the course of illness
- Is applicable early in the course of illness, in conjunction with other therapies that are intended to prolong life, such as chemotherapy or radiation therapy, and includes those investigations needed to better understand and manage distressing clinical complications

---

From: World Health Organization (2002)

---

unnecessary, expensive and potentially distressing hospital admissions and to improve the quality of life for the patient. Patients may also be referred to occupational therapies and physiotherapists, who can offer assessment, clinical care and specialist equipment to support home care. Towards the end of life, practical nursing care can be sought from agencies such as Marie Curie Cancer Care who, although predominately associated with cancer patients, have funds allocated to provide additional help during the day or night for patients with non-malignant diseases. The primary healthcare team can also refer the patient and family to more specialist palliative services if complex needs arise, for example unresolved physical symptoms or a need for more intensive psychological support.

---

**Reflection**

- Think about the last patient with a long-term condition you cared for
- How many people were involved in providing care and what roles did they perform?
- What additional personnel do you think you would need to provide effective end-of-life care?

---

## Aspects of palliative care

The holistic approach to the care of a patient and his/her carers is a key principle in palliative care requiring the successful integration of a number of different care dimensions. Each of these dimensions will require assessment on a regular and ongoing basis, with prompt treatment delivered, followed by evaluation of its effectiveness:

- Physical: managing symptoms such as pain, loss of appetite, nausea and vomiting, breathlessness, tiredness, constipation, restlessness and agitation
- Psychological: supporting the patient and those who care for them, giving time to listen and understand their concerns as well as assessing the patient for signs of depression and anxiety, which may respond to treatment
- Social: support and advice on practical and financial matters relating to the patient, their family and any other care-givers
- Spiritual: a need to explore thoughts about the meaning of life, or concerns about what happens after death. All patients are likely to have spiritual needs and for some patients this may involve completing practical things they need to do because of religious beliefs.

It is now acknowledged that patients with long-term conditions suffer with a similar symptom burden as that suffered by patients with cancer (Addington-Hall, 2008). Physical symptoms include pain, breathlessness and fatigue, also common in patients with AIDS, chronic obstructive pulmonary disease, heart disease, and renal disease (Solano et al, 2006).

Many palliative care specialists lack clinical expertise in these areas (Addington-Hall, 2008), and there is limited information on the effectiveness of treatments that were previously directed at patients with cancer. Consequently, shared care is common, with palliative care practitioners working collaboratively with disease-specific specialists, for example a heart or respiratory specialist nurses will liaise with a palliative care specialist nurse and vice versa.

The best management for patients with long-term conditions is likely to be decided on an individual patient basis, with suitable care options arrived at using local palliative care knowledge and disease-specific expertise. In many areas, a local palliative care formulary will provide useful information on the management of common symptoms.

---

**Reflection**

- Identify a patient you have cared for with a long-term condition who was moving towards the end of their life. Note their main physical problems
- Do you manage to successfully cope with these problems?
- Seek out your local palliative care formulary.

---

## Communication skills and long-term conditions

Good communication skills are fundamental to the delivery of high quality palliative care to patients and their carers, with poor communication recognized as a major factor in suboptimal palliative care (National Institute for Health and Clinical Excellence [NICE], 2004). Communication was linked to patients with long-term conditions by the WHO, who recognized the value of listening, interviewing and patient-centred communication skills as core competencies for health professionals (WHO, 2005). In the UK, the Audit Commission (1993) first highlighted the detrimental effects of poor communication skills, which left patients feeling dissatisfied with the quality of care. As a result, the *NHS Cancer Plan* (DH, 2000) recommended that communication skills be a pre-condition of qualification for professionals working within cancer care, a commitment recognized by both the General Medical and Nursing Councils (DH, 2003), and strengthened by guidance produced by NICE (2004).

The palliative phase of an illness is a sensitive and stressful time for many patients and their families. It can be difficult for health practitioners to explore the patient's and family's wishes, particularly if practitioners are inexperienced. There is evidence, however, that the majority of patients do want to be kept informed (Cox et al, 2006). Although, with regard to shared decision-making, for older patients (Cox et al, 2006) and those whose condition is worsening (Butow et al, 1997), patients may prefer their practitioners to make a higher percentage of the decisions on their behalf. The ability of patients and families to cope with life-threatening illness is shaped by many factors, including previous experiences, the degree of support available, and cultural and family traditions. Effective communication may be inhibited in these situations, particularly if health professionals lack managerial support or are inexperienced in issues related to death and dying. These difficulties are compounded with dealing with the uncertainties regarding the prognosis, which is commonplace in long-term illness (Murtagh et al, 2004).

There is now, however, a solid body of evidence that communication skills can be taught and learnt effectively in an educational environment using experiential learning techniques (Fallowfield et al, 2002; Wilkinson et al, 2008). A three-day advanced communication skills training programme (National Advanced Communication Skills Training [NCAT], 2008) attended by health professionals working within cancer care has been successfully piloted with specialist heart disease nurses (National End of Life Care Programme, 2008). In addition, there are number of helpful guidelines for broaching difficult subjects at the end of life, including von Gunten et al (2000) who suggest a seven-step approach (*Table 14.2*). Hallenbeck (2007) also suggests that, when caring for patients from different cultural backgrounds, exploring the family's prior experiences of death and dying and adding a statement of respect for the patient may be helpful.

## Bereavement care

Although inevitable, a death is a significant life event, with the loss of a loved one often causing varying degrees of psychological trauma. Emotional pain can manifest as physical symptoms with palpitations, nausea, anorexia, or even the sensation of losing a limb. As well as physical symptoms, there is an increased risk of mental health problems, such as depression and anxiety, and an increased risk of suicide, particularly among older widowers and single men losing their mothers (Worden, 2002). Comparative research studies comparing the mortality rates of control groups with the bereaved

---

**Table 14.2  Seven-step approach to communication at the end of life**

| | |
|---|---|
| Step 1 | Prepare for discussion |
| Step 2 | Establish what the patient and family already know |
| Step 3 | Determine how the information is to be handled |
| Step 4 | Deliver the information |
| Step 5 | Respond to emotions |
| Step 6 | Establish the goals for care and treatment priorities |
| Step 7 | Establish a plan |

Adapted from: von Gunten et al (2000)

---

highlight that in bereavement, men fare worse than women with the first few months being the most critical (Thomas, 2003). There is also an increased use of alcohol, tobacco, tranquilizers and hypnotics by both bereaved men and women.

The normal grieving process can be long and protracted with a 'recovery' time of two years or more being common, after which time the bereaved will have adjusted to their loss, but are often permanently altered by their experience. Gently preparing the family may be useful in improving outcomes in the bereavement period (Thomas, 2003). In fact, anticipatory grief is an acknowledged phenomenon when the patient, their spouse or other family members start the grieving process before death itself. Listening may be very helpful when visiting the bereaved, even if the time available is short. This enables the family to reflect on events, ask unanswered questions and discuss their loss, which may be psychologically helpful (El Jawahri and Prigerson, 2007). There is good evidence that children should not be excluded at this time, coping better if they are kept informed and attending funerals if they wish. Suitable strategies, however, need to be age-appropriate, as children of different ages attach different meanings to death (Kissane, 2005). Thomas (2003) makes a number of other suggestions relating to the organization of bereavement, which may be helpful to those closest to the patient (*Table 14.3*).

Occasionally, abnormal patterns of grieving occur, including chronic grief which never seems to end, delayed grief attached to a later loss, exaggerated grief linked to dysfunctional behaviour, and masked grief (Worden, 2002). In these abnormal grief reactions, specialist advice and interventions from psychological or psychiatric services may be helpful. There are a number

---

**Table 14.3 Organization of care relating to the bereaved**

- Plan to visit initially and again within three and six months of the death
- Formulate a follow-up plan in collaboration with the bereaved
- Keep good records and alert other health professionals that may come into contact with the bereaved
- Mark the anniversary
- Keep a directory, including the contact details of local bereavement counselling services, clergy, and self-help or voluntary groups that may listen, befriend and provide practical or emotional support

Adapted from: Thomas (2003)

of factors which increase the likelihood of abnormal or pathological grief. These include an ambivalent relationship with the deceased, multiple losses, previous mental illness, a sudden traumatic death, a long protracted illness, suicide, the level or perception of social support, and the inability to conduct valued rituals (Thomas, 2003). Screening is suggested as a means to identify those at greater risk of pathological grief, with assessment being undertaken on entry to a service (Kissane, 2005). Further research, however, is needed to determine the effectiveness of these tools.

Finally, it is acknowledged that health professionals often form relationships with patients and families over a long period of time. Team meetings or a reflective case study after a death may help practitioners to review their care, but also to acknowledge the death, remember the patient and off-load any residual feelings. Similarly, if appropriate some members of staff may welcome the opportunity to attend the funeral or a memorial event in order to show their respect, helping to facilitate the closure of a important episode of care.

## Specialist palliative care services

A specialist palliative care service is a term used to describe services or practitioners whose role is focused solely on patients requiring palliative care. A doctor in palliative medicine or a clinical nurse specialist in palliative care will typically undertake a distinctive training programme and will have additional qualifications specific to palliative care. A number of disciplines may be identifiable, including doctors, nurses, occupational therapists, physiotherapists, psychologists and counsellors. Within a hospice setting these core staff members may be complemented by pharmacists, dieticians, and therapy staff. Such specialist services are relatively well developed in the UK, Australia, and New Zealand, where palliative medicine was recognized as a medical specialty in late 1980s (1987 in the UK and 1988 in Canada). Unfortunately, specialist services are underdeveloped in many areas of the world, including America where palliative care skills can be lacking (Billings, 2007).

Specialist palliative care staff are most frequently based within a hospice or in units near or within an acute hospital or the community. Specialist services are designed to complement rather than replace the generalist care team, so for some patients the specialist care input may be of relatively short intervention (e.g. until a troublesome symptom has been resolved). For other patients with ongoing complex needs, specialist intervention may be required throughout the entire palliative phase of illness. This provides additional support and guidance for the patient and both professional and informal carers. In addition to providing clinical care, specialist palliative care practitioners generally have an active role in providing education for all healthcare providers and, in some cases, undertaking research studies. This helps to improve the standards of care across the healthcare community, promoting the cascade of advice on new initiatives or medications, and to help develop specialist services that are responsive to the needs of patients, their family's and other carers.

---

### Reflection

- Explore the provision of palliative care education in your area
- Attending such events on a regular basis is an important step in keeping up-to-date as new research advocates changes in medications and practice.

---

## The role of informal carers

In a community setting, the patient's family and friends become an important element of a care package, shouldering a great deal of the care that enables patients to remain at home (Milone-Nuzzo and McCorkle, 2006). The Carer's Act of 1995 sought to recognize the role of family care-givers and promoted the launch of a *Carer's National Strategy* (DH, 1999), which emphasized the shared nature of caring and the right of carers to have a life of their own outside the caring role. Although men do provide care at the end of life, the majority of care-givers are female, most commonly as the spouse or child of the dying person (Payne et al, 2008). Increasing marital breakdown and geographical mobility, as well as the opportunity for females to have paid employment outside of the home, is likely to reduce the ability of females to act in this capacity in the future (Meyers and Gray, 2001). Care-givers are also increasing likely to be elderly, with the numbers of people in the UK aged at least 85 years predicted to double from 1.1 million to 2.3 million by 2041 (Smith and Skilbeck, 2008). Frailty, multiple health problems and comorbidity will influence the ability of these care-givers to provide supportive care. Providing ongoing care, particularly in long-term illness, can be burdensome, but there is evidence that care-givers can gain satisfaction from the role if the quality of their own lives can be maintained (Smith and Skilbeck, 2008). However, evidence suggests that maintaining the quality of life of carers may be particularly difficult in rural locations (Meyers and Gray, 2001).

---

### Reflection

- Think about a palliative care patient you have nursed in a community setting
- What services were available locally to support the patient's main care-giver?
- On your next community placement, find out what services are provided for care-givers in the locality.

---

## Government end-of-life care initiatives

Research suggests that the majority of people (between 56% and 74%) express a preference to die at home (NAO, 2008), although it is acknowledged that preferences may alter as illnesses progress (NAO, 2008). Unfortunately, the majority of patients will die in an NHS hospital. The DH's *End of Life Care Strategy* suggests that 58% of patients die in hospital with 18% dying at home, 17% dying in care homes, 4% in hospices, and 3% elsewhere (DH, 2008). Some geographical variation, however, is acknowledged with statistics varying between primary care trusts (NAO, 2008). This situation is in stark contrast to the beginning of the 20th century, when dying at home was commonplace.

Variations also exist in place of death if we look at the patient's diagnosis or condition. Cancer patients are more likely to die at home or in a hospice than patients with heart and pulmonary disease, who are more likely to die in hospital (NAO, 2008). Patients with dementia are more likely to die in a care home (NAO, 2008). Although, for clinical reasons, a hospital admission may be necessary, it is recognized that a lack of timely access to community services can lead to unplanned hospital admissions (NAO, 2008). Poor information exchange between the different agencies involved can lead to inappropriate resuscitation and admission to hospital (NAO, 2008). In addition, although carer fatigue is well recognized (Thomas, 2003) there is evidence to suggest that only 29% receive an assessment of their health and social needs, with only 24% of primary care trusts being able to offer respite care to those who need it (NAO, 2008).

A lack of pre-registration training for both doctors and nurses in end-of-life care may contribute to some of these difficulties. Only 29% of doctors and 18% of nurses have received instruction in end-of-life care and although training is available in care homes, it is often not compulsory (NAO, 2008). In care homes such difficulties are compounded by the high staff turnover rates (NAO, 2008). However, there has been a renewed emphasis on end-of-life care in Government healthcare strategy, with three major initiatives designed to improve care for all patients (NICE, 2004). At least 50% of nurses and a third of doctors report having been trained in at least one of these three recommended approaches to end-of-life care, namely the Preferred Priorities for Care, the Gold Standard Framework, and the Liverpool Care Pathway (NAO, 2008).

## Preferred priorities for care

It is now considered good practice to ascertain, as the patient moves towards the end of his/her illness where he/she would prefer to die—whether this is in hospital, hospice or at home (Lugton et al, 2005). The Preferred Priorities for Care (PPC), previously the Preferred Place of Care, originated in 2003 in Lancashire and South Cumbria, where a PPC document was used to monitor the number of deaths occurring at home (Pemberton et al, 2003). When the patient's preferred place of care was recorded, their wishes were more likely to be fulfilled (Thomas, 2003). Eliciting such sensitive information from patients can be delicate and it requires confidence, good communication skills, and a sense of timing. It is also recognized that some patients may change their mind during the course of their illness, so revisiting the issues may be necessary. Opening up this sensitive subject can, however, be empowering for patients and comforting to relatives who are trying to meet the patient's wishes (Pemberton, 2004). If given by the patient, such information should be recorded and dated.

## Gold Standards Framework

The concept of teamwork in palliative care is well established and the *Gold Standards Framework* (GSF) is designed to promote better coordination, communication and delivery of palliative care in primary care (Thomas, 2003). Although it is designed for the community setting in the UK, where it has been adopted widely, it is attracting international interest (Ingleton and Seymour, 2008), although any direct benefit to patient care has yet to be proven (Walshe et al, 2008). The initial work includes identifying patients within a general practice who are most likely to die within six months. These patients are placed on a supportive care register and are the focus of discussion at regular multidisciplinary team meetings, attended by GPs, district nurses and surgery support staff. GSF care planning focuses on seven 'C's (*Table 14.4*). These act as a guide to promote communication

---

**Table 14.4 The Gold Standard Framework**

---

**Gold Standard 1: Communication**
- Regular primary healthcare team (PCHT) meetings

**Gold Standard 2: Coordination**
- Each PHCT has a nominated coordinator

**Gold Standard 3: Control of Symptoms**
- Symptoms are assessed, recorded and acted on. The patient's agenda is paramount

**Gold Standard 4: Continuity of Care Out–of-Hours**
- Practices anticipate potential need for care out-of-hours and will transfer information to reduce crises

**Gold Standard 5: Continued Learning**
- The PHCT is committed to an ongoing educational programme with a six-monthly review of training and education needs

**Gold Standard 6: Carer Support**
- Carers are supported emotionally, practically and into bereavement

**Gold Standard 7: Care of the Dying**
- Ensuring that patients are cared for appropriately at the end of life
- The use of protocols to support practice, e.g. the Liverpool Care Pathway

---

between health professionals and the patient and family. They can also provide a structure to assist the documentation of care. You will notice that the framework includes informing the out-of-hours services of the patient's condition and their preferred place of care, with the aim of ensuring the patient's final wishes are known and achieved.

Although there is evidence that using the GSF improves communication between professionals and promotes anticipatory prescribing of medication so symptoms are promptly treated (Walshe et al, 2008), there are practical issues to resolve. Establishing the likely prognosis of a patient when he/she has a long-term illness is an imprecise science. It is recognized that patients may have a longer or shorter lifespan than expected, with some living longer than six months or conversely dying unexpectedly (Addington-Hall, 2008). The advantage of the GSF, however, is that it promotes multidisciplinary dialogue, alerting members of the primary healthcare team and the surgery support staff to the fact that a patient is less well. This facilitates better communication towards the patient's desired outcomes, not only within the immediate healthcare team, but also with other agencies (e.g. services that provide care outside of normal working hours). The GSF has been adapted for care homes [GSFCH]—successful implementation requiring homes to adhere to a training programme over a one- to two-year period (Badger et al, 2009).

## Liverpool Care Pathway for the Dying Patient

The Liverpool Care Pathway for the Dying Patient (LCP) is an example of an integrated or supportive care pathway. Its clinical protocol is designed to standardize practice, promote better risk management, and encourage speedier integration of research into practice. Developed in the UK (Ellershaw and Wilkinson, 2003), it was originally designed for use in hospitals, but has evolved rapidly and is being implemented in hospital, hospices, primary care, and care homes (Ellershaw, 2007). It is designed to be used in the last few days of life and allows the cessation of medical interventions that are no longer beneficial to the patient, as well as prompting support of the patient's family and culturally-sensitive care. The pathway entails checking and documenting the patient's comfort on a regular basis, dealing promptly with a range of physical, psychosocial and spiritual issues (Ellershaw and Wilkinson, 2003) (*Table 14.5*).

The LCP documentation can be used as both an audit and an educational tool. There is evidence that it enhances the quality of documentation in a variety of care settings (hospital, nursing home, home care) and may help to decrease a patient's symptom burden, perhaps by alerting staff, although further research is needed to confirm or refute this finding (Veerbeek et al, 2008). Although initially focused on patients with cancer, recent developments aim to adapt the pathway to assist the care of patients with other conditions.

The Liverpool Care Pathway also includes clinical guidance on the treatment of the symptoms most commonly seen at the end of life in all patients, namely pain, nausea and vomiting, breathlessness, excessive respiratory secretions, restlessness and agitation.

---

### Reflection

- Is there a local champion, training event or a resource file in your current or a recent placement promoting any of the initiatives noted here?
- If so, use this opportunity to update your knowledge of practice in palliative care.

---

---

**Table 14.5 The Liverpool Care Pathway Care Goals**

**Initial assessment**

Goal 1:    Current medication assessed and non-essentials discontinued

Goal 2:    Subcutaneous medication as required, written up according to agreed guidelines

Goal 3:    Discontinue inappropriate interventions

**Psychological insight**

Goal 4:    Ability to communication in English assessed as adequate

Goal 5:    Insight into condition assessed

**Religious/spiritual support**

Goal 6:    Religious/spiritual needs assessed with patient/carer

**Communication**

Goal 7:    Identify how family/other are to be informed of patient's impending death

Goal 8:    Family/other given hospital/ hospice facilities leaflet

Goal 9:    GP practice is aware of patient's condition

**Summary**

Goal 10:  Plan of care explained and discussed with patient/family/other

Goal 11:  Family/other express understanding of plan of care

---

# Conclusion

This chapter has explored the concept of palliative care in relation to long-term conditions. The focus of palliative care has changed and now recognizes that the principles should apply to all those with a life-threatening illness, not just those with a malignancy. The provision of effective services to support palliative care requires a coordinated approach involving primary and secondary care, hospices, care homes, social services and voluntary agencies. Pathway approaches such as GCF and LCP can provide an effective way to manage and coordinate service provision. It is essential that palliative care needs are identified and met using an approach that respects patient dignity, choice and involvement. Nurses have an important role to play in all aspects of palliative care, by providing care and support, guiding patients in decision-making, and supporting relatives in times of bereavement.

Addington-Hall J (2008) Referral patterns and access to specialist palliative Care. In: Payne S, Seymour J, Ingleton C. eds, *Palliative Care Nursing: Principles and Evidence for*

*Practice*. 2nd edn.. Open University Press, Berkshire

Audit Commission (1993) *What seems to be the Matter? Communication Between Hospitals and Patients*. HMSO, London

Badger F, Clifford C, Hewison A, Thomas K (2009) An evaluation of the implementation of a programme to improve end-of-life care in nursing homes. *Palliat Med* **23**(6): 502–11

Billings JA (2007) Definitions and models of palliative care. In: Berger AM, Shuster JL, Von Roenn JH eds, *Principles and Practice of Palliative and Supportive Oncology*. 3rd edn. Lippincott Williams and Wilkins, London

Butow PN, Maclean M, Dunn SM, Tattershall MHN, Boyer MJ (1997) The dynamics of change: cancer patients' preferences for information, involvement and support. *Ann Oncol* **8**(9): 857–63

Clarke D (2004) History, gender and culture in the rise of palliative care. In: Payne S, Seymour J, Ingleton C. eds, *Palliative Care Nursing: Principles and Evidence for Practice*. Open University Press, Berkshire.

Cox A, Jenkins V, Catt S, Langridge C, Fallowfield L (2006) Information needs and experiences: An audit of UK cancer patients. *Eur J Oncol Nurs* **10**: 263–72

DH (1995) *A policy framework for commissioning cancer services: A report by the Expert Advisory Group on Cancer to the Chief Medical Officers of England and Wales*. DH, London. ref: (1995)

DH (1999) Caring about carers: a national strategy for carers. DH, London. ref: 1999

DH (2000) *The NHS Cancer plan: a plan for investment, a plan for reform*. DH, London. ref: 2000

DH (2003) *Guiding Principles relating to the commissioning and provision of communication skills training in pre-registration and undergraduate education for Healthcare Professionals*. DH, London.

DH (2004) *The NHS Improvement Plan: Putting people at the heart of public services*. DH, London. ref: 3398

DH (2008) *End of Life Care Strategy: promoting high quality care for all adults at the end of life*. DH, London. ref: 9840

Doyle D, Hanks G, Cherney NI, Calman K (2005) *Oxford textbook of palliative medicine*. 3rd edn. Oxford University Press, Oxford

Driver JA, Djoussé L, Logroscino G, Gaziano JM, Kurth T (2008) Incidence of cardiovascular disease and cancer in advanced age: prospective cohort study. *BMJ* **337**: 2521–3

El Jawahri AJ, Prigerson HG (2007) Bereavement care. In: Berger AM, Shuster JL, Von Roenn JH. eds, *Principles and Practice of Palliative Care and Supportive Oncology*. 3rd edn. Lippincott and Wilkins, London

Ellenwood AE, Jenkins JE (2007) Unbalancing the effects of chronic illness: non-traditional family therapy assessment and intervention approach. *Am J Fam Ther* **35**: 265–77

Ellershaw J, Wilkinson S (2003) Care of the dying. A pathway to excellence. Oxford University Press, Oxford.

Ellershaw J (2007) Care of the dying: what a difference an LCP makes! *Palliat Med* **21**(5): 56–8

Fallon M (2005) Palliative care in non-malignant disease. In: Doyle D, Hanks G, Cherney N, Calman K. eds, *Oxford Textbook of Palliative Medicine*. 3rd edn. Oxford University Press, Oxford

Fallowfield L, Jenkins V, Farewell V et al (2002) Efficacy of a Cancer Research UK communication skills training model for oncologists: a randomised controlled trial. *Lancet* **359**(9307): 650–6

Hallenbeck JL (2007) Cross-cultural issues. In: Berger AM, Shuster JL, Von Roenn JH. eds, *Principles and Practice of Palliative and Supportive Oncology*. 3rd edn Lippincott Williams and Wilkins, London

Higginson I (1997) Palliative and terminal care. In: Stevens A, Raftery J, Mant J, Simpson S. eds, *Health Needs Assessment: The epidemiologically based needs assessment reviews*. 2nd edn. Radcliffe Medical Press, Abingdon

Ingleton C, Seymour J (2008) Contemporary issues. In: Payne S, Seymour J, Ingleton C. eds, *Palliative Care Nursing: Principles and Evidence for Practice*. 2nd edn. Open University Press, Berkshire

Kissane DW (2005) Bereavement. In: Doyle D, Hanks G, Cherney N, Calman K. eds, *Oxford Textbook of Palliative Medicine*. 3rd edn. Oxford University Press, Oxford

Knight A (2006) Palliative care in the United Kingdom. In: Ferrell BR, Coyle N. eds, *Textbook of Palliative Nursing*. 2nd edn. Oxford university Press, Oxford

Lugton J, Frost D, Scavizzi S (2005) Communication and support in palliative care. In: Lugton J, McIntyre R. eds, *Palliative Care: The Nursing Role*. 2nd edn. Elsevier Churchill Livingstone, London

Meyers JL, Gray LN (2001) The relationships between family primary caregiver characteristics and satisfaction with hospice care, quality of life, and burden. *Oncol Nurs Forum* **28**(1): 73–82

Milone-Nuzzo P, McCorkle R (2006) Home care. In: Ferrell BR, Coyle N. eds, *Textbook of Palliative Nursing*. 2nd edn. Oxford University Press, Oxford

Murtagh FE, Preston M, Higginson I (2004) Patterns of dying: palliative care for non-malignant disease. *Clin Med* **4**(1): 39–44

NAO (2008) End of Life Care. http://tinyurl.com/bs8o8t (accessed 15 December 2009)

National End of Life Care Programme (2008) Advanced communication skills pilot training course. http://tinyurl.com/ygl4uv5 (accessed 15 November 2009)

NCAT (2008) National advanced communication skills training programme for senior health care professional in cancer care. www.connected.nhs.uk (accessed 15 November 2009)

NICE (2004) Improving supportive and palliative care for adults with cancer. http://

guidance.nice.org.uk/CSGSP (accessed 15 November 2009)

Payne S, Seymour J, Ingleton C (2008) Introduction. In: Payne S, Seymour J, Ingleton C. eds, *Palliative Care Nursing: Principles and Evidence for Practice*. 2nd edn. Open University Press, Berkshire

Pemberton C, Storey L, Howard A (2003) The Preferred Place of Care document: an opportunity for communication. *Int J Palliat Nurs* **9**(10): 439–41

Pemberton C (2004) *Understanding the preferred place of care document: its place in practice*. RCN Palliative Care Nursing Group, London

Saunders CM (2005) Foreword. In: Doyle D, Hanks G, Cherney N, Calman K. eds, *Oxford Textbook of Palliative Medicine*. 3rd edn. Oxford University Press, Oxford

Smith P, Skilbeck J (2008) Working with family care-givers in a palliative setting. In: Payne S, Seymour J, Ingleton C. eds, *Palliative Care Nursing: Principles and Evidence for Practice*. 2nd edn. Open University Press, Berkshire

Solano JP, Gomes B, Higginson IJ (2006) A comparison of symptom prevalence in far advanced cancer, AIDS, heart disease, chronic obstructive pulmonary disease and renal disease. *J Pain Symptom Manage* **31**(1): 58–69

Thomas K (2003) *Caring for the Dying at Home: Companions on a journey*. Radcliffe Medical Press, Oxon

Veerbeek L, van Zuylen L, Swart SJ et al (2008) The effect of the Liverpool Care Pathway for the dying: a multi-centre study. *Palliat Med* **22**(2): 145–51

von Gunten CF, Ferris FD, Emanuel LL (2000) The patient-physician relationship. Ensuring competency in end-of-life care: communication and relational skills. *JAMA* **284**(23): 3051–7

Walshe C, Caress A, Chew-Graham C, Todd C (2008) Implementation and impact of the Gold Standards Framework in community palliative care: a qualitative study of three primary care trusts. Palliat Med 22(6): 736–43

Wilkinson S, Perry R, Blanchard K, Linsell L (2008) Effectiveness of a three-day communication skills course in changing nurses' communication skills with cancer/palliative care patients: a randomised controlled trial. *Palliat Med* **22**(4): 365–75

Worden JW (2002) Bereavement care. In: Berger AM, Portenoy RK, Weissman DE. eds, *Principles and Practice of Palliative and Supportive Oncology*. 2nd edn. Lippincott Williams and Wilkins, London

WHO (2002) Definition of Palliative Care. www.who.int/cancer/palliative/definition/en/ (accessed 15 November 2009)

WHO (2005) Preparing a Health Care Workforce for the 21st Century: The Challenge of Chronic Conditions. http://tinyurl.com/yj3pwjf (accessed 15 December 2009)

WHO (2009) Definition of Palliative Care. http://tinyurl.com/5228js (accessed 15 December 2009)

# Useful websites

*Liverpool Care Pathway: www.mcpcil.org.uk/liverpool-care-pathway/index.htm*

*Gold Standard Framework: www.goldstandardsframework.nhs.uk/*

*Preferred Priorities for Care: www.endoflifecareforadults.nhs.uk/eolc/CS310.htm*

*End of Life Programme: www.endoflifecareforadults.nhs.uk/*

# CHAPTER 15

# Collaborative working

*Helen McVeigh*

Providing effective health care to support individuals with a long-term condition requires a coordinated approach that recognizes the multi-professional nature of service provision. The Nursing and Midwifery Council (NMC) recognizes the need for effective collaboration and the importance of enabling individuals to access relevant health and social care, and support (NMC, 2008).

This chapter explores some of the different services, agencies and care providers who may offer support to those with chronic conditions. It explores the concept of collaboration and identifies the opportunities and challenges that influence effective inter-professional working.

By reading this chapter, and through personal reflection, the following learning outcomes can be achieved:

*   An understanding of the variety and scope of the different service providers
*   An awareness of the barriers to effective collaboration
*   An awareness of strategies which can facilitate effective team working.

## Service provision

The patient with a long-term condition may benefit from support and/or intervention from a number of services. For the majority of patients, service provision will originate and terminate in primary care (Department of Health [DH], 2002). The Government clearly highlights a significant position and role for primary care services in meeting these needs (DH, 2006; 2008a, 2008b).

The services that are available to support independent living are sourced from a wide range of providers that include statutory, voluntary, and private sector agencies, and informal care (*Table 15.1*).

**Table 15.1 Service provision**

| Agency | Service example |
|---|---|
| Statutory agencies | Health services |
| | Social services |
| | Emergency services |
| Voluntary agencies | Help the Aged |
| | Samaritans |
| Charitable organizations | NSPCC |
| | Age Concern |
| | British Red Cross |
| Patient groups | Multiple Sclerosis Society |
| Mutual aid societies | Royal British Legion |
| Private health care | BUPA |
| | Residential homes |
| | Nursing homes |
| Informal care | Family members |
| | Neighbours/friends |

## Statutory services

These services are provided/financed by the state, and include health and social care. They are driven by Government policies—provision is often influenced by changes in the political agenda.

## Private sector

These services are located in a competitive market and generally seek to make a profit. Charges are made for the services provided. They include private hospitals, and residential and nursing homes.

In some instances, the private sector works jointly with the public sector. By using private sector funding, public and private sector partnerships can work together in cooperation to provide services and facilities; Local Improvement Finance Trust (LIFT) and Private Finance Initiatives (PFIs) are examples of this. LIFT was a £1 billion programme focused on inner-city areas, where health needs are the greatest, to build new primary care facilities across England (DH, 2009a). The private sector funds the building/refurbishment of hospital or primary care premises. The private sector then leases the accommodation to the healthcare providers, typically under 25–30 year contracts. The private sector may also provide maintenance and support services throughout this time (DH, 2009a). These partnerships can be beneficial; the advantages are that projects can be often be completed quicker than in the public sector and the private sector may be able to reduce costs in the design, construction and maintenance of facilities. There are potential limitations, however; 25–30 year contracts may not be flexible enough to respond to changes in the healthcare sector and partnership working may suffer in an environment with both private and public employers.

## Social enterprise

Social enterprise organizations operate along business lines. They are non-profit making and any profit is reinvested for the benefit of the community or in innovative service developments. Their aims include encouraging staff, patients and service users to be involved in designing the services delivered (DH, 2006; 2009b). There are opportunities for those working within statutory provision to identify, organize and set up service provision within the social enterprise scheme. Examples of healthcare services set up include Local Care Direct and Open Door.

## Voluntary organizations

These are non-statutory bodies ranging from self-help groups to large charitable foundations. They do not seek to make a profit. Some will have charitable status and are registered as charities. They may pay people to work for them, but many rely on unpaid volunteers.

## Volunteers

A wide range of activities and tasks may be carried out by volunteers for individuals in their own homes. Data gathered by the charity Community Service Volunteers suggests that volunteers give over 88 million hours every year (Davis Smith, 1998). Volunteer contributions can help individuals to increase and/or maintain their independence and improve the quality of life for those they support (Bowers et al, 2006).

## Informal care

Many individuals rely on the help of families, neighbours and friends to provide care. Many of these informal carers spend a significant proportion of their lives providing unpaid support to family or friends. It is estimated that there are approximately six million informal carers in the UK, and around half will be aged 50–64 years (Mooney et al, 2002).

**Reflection**

- Identify a patient you have nursed who has a long-term condition
- What services other than statutory healthcare provision do they access?

Within service provision, a variety of different skills and expertise are provided by a wide range of professionals, including:

- Specialist nurses
- Allied health professionals—chiropody, physiotherapy, occupational therapy
- Social workers
- Home carers
- Counsellors
- Expert patients
- Language translators.

Expertise and skill may be unique to a particular service provider, although there are many areas which will inevitably overlap between individual services, particularly in the provision of health and social care. Nurses need to be aware that services can complement each other and that non-statutory agencies may be able to offer unique expertise or support (Ward, 2001). Of particular note is the increasing role that voluntary agencies and charities now play in service provision. The Government has recognized the importance and value of their potential (DH, 2005), and actively encourages their participation and inclusion in service provision. They can be ideally placed to deliver services to local communities and often have a specific awareness of the needs and wishes of their service users (Russell, 2006). Nurses may feel less than confident in routinely using this type of service provision, owing to concerns around levels of accountability, codes of practice, and how they are organized and governed (Ward, 2001). The unpredictable nature of their sources of income (reliance on grants or donations), particularly with smaller charities, may also lead the professional to question their ongoing sustainability as part of a care package. However, the value of the voluntary sector should not be underestimated as input can positively influence quality of life for patients. Although not governed by professional bodies, voluntary agencies are held responsible for the services they provide, charitable organizations are regulated by the Charity Commission, and all are accountable to their funders, trustees and clients (Ward, 2001; Cook, 2008). Nurses should be prepared to consider how these resources can be effectively incorporated into meeting the needs of patients.

The numbers of different people and agencies who may be involved in care delivery highlights the need for services to communicate effectively and strive for efficient collaboration. Agencies all too frequently work independently and fail to communicate and coordinate with others, which can result in duplication of, or gaps in, service provision (Doyle, 2008), which will inevitably impact on patient outcomes. The nurse in primary care is in a key position to advise, direct or refer patients to additional service providers and therefore, should be aware of the scope, range and choices available.

## Collaboration

Historically, the structure and function of health and social care services were based on uni-professional cultures, working alongside but not necessarily in partnership with each other. However, in recent years there has been a significant shift to emphasize the value and importance of inter-professional collaboration. The drive to modernize the NHS was based on fundamental principles highlighting the need to provide a coordinated service and encourage collaborative working (DH, 2000), while also acknowledging that the needs of the patient should be maintained at the forefront of care. Service user consultation identified that people want seamless, proactive and integrated services tailored to their needs (DH, 2008c). The need to improve collaboration, particularly between health and social care, is increasingly emphasized in national policy (DH, 2006; 2008a). Effective care provision should be about considering the workforce as teams of people, rather than individual professions, with the aim of reducing professional tribalism (DH, 2000). Ensuring effective and high quality care requires the crossing and dismantling of professional boundaries (Wakefield et al, 2003). The overall emphasis should be on coordinated service provision, founded on common aims, equal partnerships, negotiation and shared decision-making.

It is equally important to remember that the patient and his/her family are a fundamental part of this process. Effective service provision can only be implemented through a negotiated partnership that recognizes patient choice in identifying agreed outcomes and the decisions made:

- Collaboration: Active participation between two or more people to achieve a common goal
- Inter-professional: A group with distinct disciplinary training working together for a common purpose, who make different yet complementary contributions to patient care.

---

**Table 15.2 The benefits of collaboration**

---

- High standards of care
- Continuity of care
- Holistic care provision
- Pooled skills/knowledge and abilities
- Improved cost-effectiveness
- Improved patient outcomes
- Improved communication
- Reduce duplication
- Shared goals/solidarity
- Appropriate use of specialist skill
- Shared learning
- Mutual respect between professions/professionals

---

Collaboration requires more than just coordination or cooperation with other service providers. Ideally, it should involve joint planning, shared resources and joint resource management. True collaboration takes place through shared understanding, open communication, mutual trust and tolerance of differing viewpoints. The benefits of collaborative working can be seen from organizational, professional and patient perspectives (Ward, 2001). *Table 15.2* highlights the main benefits of a collaborative approach.

While it is evident that multi-professional service provision is often necessary to effectively meet the needs of patients with long-term conditions, and that a collaborative approach should be central to providing high quality care and improving patient outcomes, it is widely recognized that there are many barriers to effective inter-professional working (*Table 15.3*). By recognizing the factors which influence how well we collaborate with other professions, and identifying how we can overcome these, nurses can work towards ensuring service provision becomes truly seamless and patient-centred.

---

**Reflection**

- Consider your working environment and the team you work with
- How well do you communicate with other professionals?
- What prevents effective collaboration in your team?

---

---

**Table 15.3 Barriers to inter-professional collaboration**

---

- Poor communication
- Issues around information sharing and confidentiality
- Duplication of services/paperwork
- Fragmented teams
- Fear of loss of professional identity
- Fear of change
- Limited knowledge and understanding of the roles of others
- Professional rivalry/tribalism
- Different management structures and hierarchies
- Different funding/resources
- Complex multi-professional teams
- Different workplace bases

---

## Teamwork

Good teamwork is essential for effective service delivery. As a nurse, it is important to recognize the factors that enable a team to function effectively. In order to facilitate good team working, it is useful to reflect on your role and the team that you work in:

- Do you have a clear understanding of your role within the team?
- Do you feel valued and part of the team?
- Is the team functioning efficiently?
- Does the team have clear aims, objectives and direction?
- What factors make this a good team?

Identifying the strengths and weaknesses of your own team can help to establish where difficulties may arise in liaison and collaboration with others. It is possible to draw some parallels between the essentials of what makes a successful team and the factors which will enable good inter-professional collaboration (*Table 15.4*). The strengths of the multi-professional team may lie in its ability to look at issues from differing perspectives and to offer more creative or resourceful solutions to problems.

It is important to remember that care should remain patient-focused. By using a patient-directed approach, it is possible for the foundation of inter-professional teamwork to be built on shared aims and objectives. This can foster a collective responsibility for the services delivered.

---

**Table 15.4 What makes a successful team?**

---

- Good communication
- Common objectives/shared vision
- Good leadership
- Involvement of all members
- Mutual trust
- Role identity/clarity
- Supportive culture
- Appropriate skills/expertise
- Appropriate training
- Standards
- Openness

---

Working towards shared aims requires an understanding of the roles and responsibilities of others. There is often a lack of clarity both within and between teams with regard to who should provide what and where the service boundaries lie (Sloper, 2004). If we are unaware of the role and responsibilities others play in the delivery of care, there are inherent dangers of duplicating provision (Thomas and While, 2007), of failure to offer patients truly informed choices and ultimately, poorer patient outcomes. The patient with a long-term condition may have multiple service providers. A lack of role awareness will impact negatively on the relationship we develop with our patient and subsequently on the confidence they may have in us.

> *'If we do not understand each other's roles how can we expect a patient to do so?'*
>
> *Holland (2004: 228)*

An increased understanding of the role of others can potentially reduce professional rivalry and encourage mutual respect and trust. Therefore, effective collaboration will require professionals to develop confidence in both their own role and its boundaries, and also to develop an awareness, respect and understanding of others (Davies and Northway, 2001; Ward, 2001).

### Communication

One of the primary problems in the facilitation of effective inter-professional collaboration is the issue of effective communication. Nursing expertise is underpinned by the necessity for good communication skills. While we develop excellent communication skills in our interaction with patients and within nursing teams, this does not often duplicate in our interaction with other professions or outside our immediate working environment. Media reports note that poor communication is frequently the root cause of complaints in health care. Nurses should recognize that good communication between professionals both within professions and multi-professionally is paramount to effective care provision.

The problem of poor communication has been highlighted by high profile cases, such as those of Victoria Climbié and Baby P, where the lack of effective communication across professional groups and services were cited as the main cause of inefficiency (Wakefield et al, 2003; Department for Children Schools and Families, 2009). The issue of effective communication between multiple service providers has been addressed in some part by recent Government initiatives to implement coordinated care plans and the use of a single assessment process (SAP) or common assessment framework (CAF) (DH, 2001; 2003; 2009c).

SAP and CAF focus on the use of one document and one process of assessment throughout all services. The focus is on person-centred holistic assessment, which increases efficiency and can improve information sharing (Centre for Policy on Ageing, 2009). The aim is to facilitate effective care delivery within multidisciplinary teams, while addressing the issue of effectively managing agency boundaries (Leaver, 2004). This can improve the patient experience when negotiating the maze of service providers they may come in to contact with. The literature highlights the case of one patient who had 37 different providers, all with differing expectations, but requiring much duplicated information (Howkins and Thornton, 2003). Personalized care-planning is part of this process. All the information required by different providers should be located in one overarching care plan. For patients with complex needs and care provision, a named lead professional will be identified. This addresses the issue that patients sometimes do not know who to contact when faced with a multitude of services and professionals. Thomas and While (2007) take a conceptual view, suggesting that multi-professional care provision can be viewed as a railway network where it is essential that passengers (patients) have clear maps that reveal where the routes intersect, and timetables for when they can travel, in order to successfully negotiate the system. Sharing documentation can be seen as good practice (Miers and Pollard, 2009). For patients, there are clear benefits in the elimination of confusion and continuity of care provision; and for professionals, in reducing the duplication of paperwork, providing coordinated holistic care, and potential savings in resources and staff requirements (Freeth, 2001). Streamlining assessment supports the aim to maintain services that are led by the needs of clients/patients, rather than the reverse.

Effective communication is not reliant on sound methods of assessment alone. It also requires improved pathways of communication and effective liaison between professionals that recognizes the limitations and boundaries of the professions and teams we work with. Identifying appropriate methods of communication that can cross professional and geographical boundaries, and the use of common language across professions, is important. Good communication is often hampered by services working from different bases, differing shift patterns, and different hours of service provision. The efficient use of technology (e-mail, internet, virtual conferencing) can increase the potential for effective communication between teams (Marquis and Huston, 2009), particularly when teams are not co-located. It is clear that nurses need to develop methods of efficient communication both internally within their team, and externally to facilitate effective collaboration.

Regular multi-professional team meetings, joint training and activities can promote inter-professional team-building. There are already established moves towards incorporating an inter-professional focus in many of the health professions education programmes; however, it is important to recognize that the reality needs to be more than simply professionals learning common content side-by-side, but should include a significant emphasis on team working and interaction. True inter-professional education should focus on understanding roles and learning from and about each other to improve collaboration and quality of care (Holland, 2002; Cullen et al, 2003). Introducing inter-professional education strategies early in programmes of education might prevent attitudes and professional barriers from developing and may address the negative stereotyping that frequently hinders inter-professional collaboration.

Effective inter-professional team working and communication is also influenced by the size of organizations (Miers and Pollard, 2009). The NHS and social services are large and complex organizations, and multiple lines of management and accountability will inevitably create barriers and challenges (Bigger, 2004). The DH (2008a) suggests we should be moving towards integrated working between health and social care, which can include true multidisciplinary teams, co-located and aligned to one organization. Recent service developments have seen the emergence of intermediate care services, for example rapid access, hospital-at-home and hospice-at-home teams. These service developments are supported by changes to general practice working outlined in the General Medical Services contract, which increases the opportunity for better networking within the multidisciplinary and multi-agency teams, and encourages cross–practice activity to meet patient need (White et al, 2004). These services coordinate and provide care and support to patients, incorporating both health and social service sectors, with the fundamental aim of maintaining individuals within the home environment. These can be viewed as good examples of partnership working, 'organising services around patients and not people around services' (DH, 2008a: 43), and bringing together different agencies with a common goal.

Changing demographics and increasing demands on health care to manage long-term conditions, as well as the emphasis on care provision closer to home, means that the future direction for service provision will increasingly focus on effective partnership working. Nurses are increasingly encouraged to take part in the planning and development of services. The challenge of providing high quality, individualized care and flexible, responsive services in the future may rely on our ability to identify, plan and coordinate innovative and effective ways of working in partnership with others.

## Case history I

Primrose is a 68-year-old spinster. She has one nephew who visits occasionally, but no other family support. She lives in a second floor warden-controlled flat. She suffered a stroke four weeks ago and is currently an inpatient on the rehabilitation ward of the local community hospital. Following intensive rehabilitation, she is now ready for discharge home. The stroke has left her with a profound left-sided weakness. She is able to stand and take one or two steps with the aid of a walking frame, but is rather unsteady and has lost a lot of confidence in her abilities. Before the stroke she was very independent—she had always done her own cooking, cleaning and shopping. She has a good network of friends and is quite outgoing. She enjoys meeting up with her friends to go on organized day trips and they regularly attend the weekly lunch club and the local church. Primrose is desperate to get home to her flat and her friends, but she is worried about how she will cope.

Primrose would benefit from a home assessment before her discharge from hospital. This should be a joint assessment involving all agencies and services who might be involved in her ongoing care. Examples of service provision she might benefit from include:

- Equipment provision or adaptions to her flat: Red Cross or local provider
- Intensive support in first few weeks: Community matron, intermediate care team
- Social care package to meet hygiene needs: Social worker, home care
- Ongoing rehabilitation: Physiotherapist, occupational therapist, speech and language therapist

- Basic needs (e.g. food): Meals on wheels, shopping (friends, home care, internet)
- Social and psychological needs: Voluntary groups (e.g. Age Concern), community transport, befriending service
- Safety and Security: Warden, friends and neighbours, community alarm
- Health promotion: Practice/district nurse, pharmacy.

Primrose would need a coordinated package of care and she should be involved in the decision-making process. Shared assessment and an agreed individualized patient-held care plan are important. For Primrose, coming to terms with a loss of independence is going to be challenging, knowing who, what and when with regard to her care is paramount to give her back some control and choice in improving her quality of life.

---

### Reflection

- Look at the second case history
- What services would be helpful in this case?
- Consider the service provision for this case. How could this best be coordinated to provide effective care?

---

## Case history 2

Sarah Johnson is 76 years old and Cyril Johnson is 78 years old. Sarah and Cyril have been married for 55 years, and live in a small terraced house in the city centre. They have two daughters, both married and in full-time employment. Both children are very supportive of their parents. They have organized a rota to visit on alternate days in the evening after work, and undertake all the shopping and cleaning for them. Sarah has rheumatoid arthritis, which was diagnosed when she was 45 years old. Sarah has very limited mobility, is unable to weight bear, and spends most of the day in her wheelchair. The house was adapted some years ago and there is a ceiling hoist, walk-in shower room and a variable height bed. Sarah sleeps in the converted front room downstairs. Cyril has been the main carer for Sarah over the last 10 years, since she became less mobile. He has home care to help him get Sarah out of bed in the morning, and the family help him in the evening. Cyril and Sarah rarely leave the house unless it is a special family occasion. Cyril is a diabetic. He was diagnosed 15 years ago and has been well controlled on insulin therapy for the last five years. He administers his own insulin, and is knowledgeable about his diabetes, the importance of a diabetic diet and monitoring his blood glucose levels. Recently, he has had elevated blood glucose levels and on one occasion he had a hypoglycaemic episode. His practice nurse is concerned that his $HbA_{1C}$ level is elevated. Cyril has admitted that his eyesight is not as good as it used to be. The family are becoming concerned that Cyril can no longer cope with managing his own health and caring for Sarah. Cyril insists that 'he has managed up to now and that all he needs is some new glasses', and that 'we have been together for 55 years and nobody is putting us in a home now'.

## Conclusion

This chapter has looked at the nature of service provision to meet the needs of individuals with a long-term condition. Service provision may be from statutory, private, voluntary or informal sources, and will frequently rely on a coordinated approach using a range of different sources. The focus of inter-professional working should remain patient-centred and patient involvement is an important element of this process. As a nurse it is important to be aware of which services and agencies are available in order to provide patients with advice, support and care that reflects an informed choice of service provision. Quality care is reliant on working well together. A collaborative approach is fundamental to effective care and improved patient outcomes. Collaboration can have benefits for service users, professionals and organizations. Good communication and skilled teamwork across professional boundaries will result in coordinated and proactive services that improve patient outcomes and meet the needs of the individual and the community.

Bigger M (2004) The link between commissioning and teamwork within primary care. *Journal of Community Nursing*: 4–11

Bowers H, Macadam A, Patel M, Smith C (2006) Making a difference through volunteering: The impact of volunteers who support and care for people at home. http://tinyurl.com/yhoewgks. (accessed 24 November 2009)

Centre for Policy on Ageing (2009) The Common Assessment Framework. http://tinyurl.com/yd7qdbl (accessed 24 November 2009)

Cook R (2008) Nursing leadership and management in third-sector organisations. *Nurs Manag* 15(7): 24–9

Cullen L, Fraser D, Symonds I (2003) Strategies for interprofessional education: the Interprofessional Team Objective Structured Clinical Examination for midwifery and medical students. *Nurse Educ Today* **23**(6):427–33

Davies D, Northway R (2001) Collaboration in primary care. *Journal of Community Nursing*: 14–8

Davis Smith J (1998) *The 1997 National Survey of Volunteering*. National Centre for Volunteering, London

Department for Children Schools and Families (2009) Safeguarding the Young and Vulnerable: The Joint Chief Inspectors' recommendations and the Government's responses one year on. http://tinyurl.com/lmmclx (accessed 24 November 2009)

DH (2000) The NHS Plan: a plan for investment, a plan for reform. http://tinyurl.com/2phr42 (accessed 24 November 2009)

DH (2001) *National Service Framework for Older People*. DH, London. ref: 2001

DH (2002) *Liberating the talents: Helping primary care trusts and nurses to deliver the NHS Plan*. DH, London. ref: 2002

DH (2003) *Single Assessment Process for Older People: The accreditation process for off-the-shelf assessment tools*. DH, London. ref: 2003

DH (2005) *National Strategic Partnership Forum—Statement of Purpose*. DH, London. ref: 5285

DH (2006) Our Health, Our Care, Our Say. http://tinyurl.com/yvkmdx (accessed 24 November 2009)

DH (2008a) *High quality care for all: NHS Next Stage Review final report*. DH, London. ref: 10106

DH (2008b) *NHS Next Stage Review: Our vision for primary and community care*. DH, London. ref: 10096

DH (2008c) *Long term conditions compendium of information*. DH, London. ref: 8734

DH (2009a) NHS LIFT FAQ. http://tinyurl.com/yks7y5u (accessed 24 November 2009)

DH (2009b) Social enterprise. http://tinyurl.com/y9ouw8k (accessed 24 November 2009)

DH (2009c) *Common Assessment Framework for Adults. a consultation on proposals to improve information sharing around multi-disciplinary assessment and care planning*. DH, London. ref: 11096

Doyle J (2008) Barriers and facilitators of multidisciplinary team working: a review. *Paediatr Nurs* **20**(2): 26–9

Freeth D (2001) Sustaining interprofessional collaboration. *J Interprof Care* **15**(1): 37–46

Holland K (2002) Inter-professional education and practice: the role of the teacher/facilitator. *Nurse Educ Pract* **2**(4): 221–2

Holland K (2004) Inter-professional working and learning for integrated health and social care services. *Nurse Educ Pract* **4**(4): 228–9

Howkins E, Thornton C (2003) Liberating the talents: whose talents and for what purpose? *J Nurs Manag* **11**(4): 219–20

Leaver R (2004) The single assessment process. *Prof Nurse* **19**(9): 513

Marquis B, Huston C (2009) *Leadership Roles and Management Functions in Nursing; Theory and Application.* 6th edn. Lippincott Williams and Wilkins, Philadelphia

Miers M, Pollard K (2009) The role of nurses in interprofessional health and social care teams. *Nurs Manag* **15**(9): 30–5

Mooney A, Statham J, Simon A (2002) Informal Care and Work after 50. Joseph Rowntree Foundation. http://tinyurl.com/y9ue4p9 (accessed 24 November 2009)

NMC (2008) The Code: Standards of conduct, performance and ethics for nurses and midwives. http://tinyurl.com/6kdup6 (accessed 24 November 2009)

Russell V (2006) Voluntary sector knows best how to involve service users. *Public Finance London*: 24–30 November

Sloper P (2004) Facilitators and barriers for co-ordinated multi-agency services. *Child Care Health Dev* **30**(6): 571–80

Thomas P, While A (2007) Should nurses be leaders of integrated health care? *J Nurs Manag* **15**(6): 643–8

Wakefield A, Furber C, Boggis A, Sutton A, Cooke S (2003) Promoting interdisciplinarity through educational initiative: a qualitative evaluation. *Nurse Educ Pract* **3**(4): 195–203

Ward D (2001) Working with non-statutory agencies. *Journal of Community Nursing*: 4–11

White E, Singer R, McQuarrie R (2004) An opportunity for community nurses? *Community Pract* **77**(4): 129–30

# Further information

*Local Care Direct: www.localcaredirect.org/index.php5*

*Open Door: www.opendooronline.org*

# CHAPTER 16

# Using technology to manage health care

*Helen McVeigh*

This chapter explores the challenge of managing long-term conditions in the 21$^{st}$ century. It is recognized that changing demographics and an increasing burden on health care from chronic disease will raise significant challenges to the provision of care in the future. The fundamental aims of quality health care for those with long-term conditions are to add life to years as well as years to life (Department of Health [DH], 2008a). Technological advances in modern society mean that there are a variety of ways in which to enable individuals to remain in their own homes for as long as possible, and to enjoy a better quality of life regardless of any chronic condition.

This chapter explores the types of technology available and considers the advantages and disadvantages of using them. Reading this chapter and reflecting on your own experiences should enable you to achieve the following learning outcomes:

* An understanding of the challenges facing healthcare provision in the future
* An awareness of the technology available to support the provision of health care for individuals with a long-term condition
* An awareness of the benefits and disadvantages of using technology to support patients.

## Background

There are over 15 million people in England living with a long-term condition. It is projected that by 2025 these numbers will have risen by around 3 million to somewhere in excess of 18 million people (DH, 2008a). Factors influencing the rise in these figures include increasing life expectancy (although not necessarily a healthy life) and the increased means to keep people in ill-health living for longer.

The main challenge for health professionals should be to reduce the burden of disease and maintain an acceptable quality of life for those living with long-term conditions. It is acknowledged that current healthcare initiatives are aimed at preventive strategies with long-term aims to reduce the future burden of preventable conditions. While it is important that health education and promotion continue to target these issues, the reality is that large numbers of people are already suffering from a preventable condition and are likely to live to old age. In addition, a great amount of people may already have the increased risk factors for developing conditions such as coronary heart disease, chronic obstructive pulmonary disease, and diabetes in the future. This may be compounded by additional challenges relating to current lifestyle factors, such as obesity and levels of alcohol consumption, the effect of which on chronic disease patterns may be greater than anticipated.

As well as increasing levels of chronic disease, there have been societal changes. Individuals have greater expectations of living for longer and of having a better quality of life. Modern living has seen a greater geographical mobility with resultant fragmentation of family groups. As a consequence, there are increasing numbers of older people who live alone and who may lack the available support from family members to remain independent. The increased burden of coping with this level of chronic disease within a finite health system means there is a need to explore alternative methods and solutions of ensuring individuals living with a long-term condition can do so with a level of care or support that meets their needs.

The changing profile of health and disease in the UK has highlighted that there is a need for more creative solutions to meet increasing demand. In order to meet the needs of individuals, the Government recognizes that care should be holistic and personalized. *Our Health, Our Care, Our Say* (DH, 2006) suggests that by 2010 everyone with a long-term condition should be offered an individualized care plan. This commitment is reiterated in Lord Darzi's report, *High Quality Care for All* (DH, 2008b), which notes that care plans should be personalized, negotiated, agreed with the individual, and regularly reviewed. This recognizes that patients should be equipped with the knowledge, support and information to make truly informed choices with regard to their ongoing management and support. These documents also indicate that there is a role for assistive technology in achieving these aims. Enabling individuals to remain independent for as long as possible requires a coordinated approach which incorporates an element of self-care and management. Recognition of the value of self-care in the ongoing management of long-term conditions is echoed in the *Common Core Principles to Support Self Care* (Skills for Health, 2008), principle 5, which notes that assisted self-care may include the provision of support to enable individuals to use the appropriate technology. *Your Health, Your Way* (DH, 2009a) highlights assistive technology as one of the key tools for delivering effective support for self-care. This underlines an expectation that the professional, whether this is health or social care, should ensure that appropriate equipment and devices are discussed and that their availability, provision and ongoing support to use them is provided (Skills for Health, 2008).

Using assistive technology is supported by DH funding as part of a commitment to modernize care services. In 2006, local authorities were awarded an £80 million preventive technology grant over two years to set up the infrastructure to support telecare (DH, 2005). The Government has also invested in the Whole System Demonstrator Programme, a two-year project started in May 2008 in three pilot sites across the UK (Cornwall, Kent and Newham) (Whole System Demonstrator Action Network, 2009). This project aims to examine the effect of technology on patient experience, quality of life, emergency admission rates, and assess its impact on primary care.

## Using the technology

The use of technological equipment is integrated within all walks of life. Expectations have risen and our society is increasingly reliant on its use. Mobile phones, home computers and internet shopping, all of which were the stuff of science fiction just a few decades ago, are now an everyday normality. It is not surprising, therefore, that this transformation has extended into the healthcare arena. It is estimated that between 50–80% of adults will use the internet to access health information (Antai-Otong, 2007). The use of technology to support and enable independent living is not entirely new either. Health professionals are familiar with the provision of equipment to elderly or vulnerable adults, such as community alarms, which have been used for many years as a valuable device. The increasing availability and range of technology means it is important that its provision is individualized, based on need, accessible and equitable to all that would benefit from it (DH, 2005). Technology can be viewed as supporting patients' needs on a variety of levels (Liddell et al, 2008):

* Information and education
* Social inclusion and connectivity

- Diagnosis and consultation
- Individual choice
- Behavioural modification and support
- Care and lifestyle monitoring.

## Definitions

There is a variety of terminology associated with technology to support health care and independent living. It is useful to explore the definitions for the different types of technology available:

- *Assistive technology*. This is any product or service designed to enable independence for people with disabilities and those who are older. It is often used as a general term for a variety of health-related technologies
- *e-health*. Health services, information or education delivered or enhanced through the internet and related technologies
- *Telecare*. The continuous, automatic and remote monitoring of real-time emergencies and lifestyle changes in order to manage the risks associated with independent living. For example, electronic aids and sensors that make the home environment safer and enable individuals to continue to live at home independently
- *Telehealth*. The delivery of health care at a distance, using electronic means of communication, usually from patient to clinician. For example, electronic sensors or equipment used to monitor an individuals' health in their own home (vital signs, e.g. blood pressure, blood glucose levels, blood oxygen levels). Data is transmitted electronically to health professionals
- *Telemedicine*. The delivery of health care or sharing of clinical information from separate geographical locations using electronic means of communication—usually from one professional to another. For example, a GP undertaking an electrocardiogram on a patient suspected of heart disease and transfer of that data to a specialist clinician for discussion (Liddell et al, 2008; DH Care Networks, 2009).

*Table 16.1* illustrates some examples of the types of technology available.

## Table 16.1 Examples of assistive technology

**e-health**
- Electronic health records
- Common Assessment Framework
- Text reminders for appointments

**Assistive technology stand-alone devices**
- Electronic medication dispenser/intelligent pill dispenser/medication alert reminders
- Memory or picture phone
- Night light with motion sensor
- Pressure plugs used in baths and sinks to prevent flooding
- Vibrating door alert

**Telecare equipment**
- Equipment is linked to a control centre. Once triggered, a signal is received by the control centre. Action is taken in response to a trigger and is agreed by the client/patient and his/her family
- Activity monitoring—triggered as person moves around the house
- Bed or chair occupancy detector
- Extreme heat sensor (e.g. if cooker left on)
- Falls detector
- Gas sensor with shut off valve
- Pendant alarm/panic alarm/bogus caller
- Property exit sensor

**Telehealth equipment**
Computerized systems for monitoring vital signs. Data is monitored and collected in a patients' home and this is relayed back to a central web-based secure server, which can only be accessed by authorized personnel. Readings are taken by the individual (or family member) and are transmitted electronically to health professionals (GP, community matron, and nurse). Equipment may be wireless and often requires a broadband connection

### Reflection

- Think about patients you have met.
- What types of technology have you seen used to support independent living?

The value of using technology can be seen from both economic and quality of life perspectives. These benefits link to better clinical outcomes for the patient, an improved patient experience and cost-effectiveness for healthcare provision (Barlow et al, 2007; Joint Improvement Team, 2008; Liddell et al, 2008). The potential benefits include (DH, 2005):

* Contributing to the care and support of individuals with long-term conditions
* Increasing choice and independence
* Reducing the burden on informal carers
* Reducing admissions to residential and nursing homes
* Reducing emergency hospital admissions
* Reducing accidents and falls in the elderly
* Supporting earlier hospital discharges and intermediate care
* Contributing to the development of preventive services
* Helping those who wish to die at home to do so
* Improved use of resources.

Assistive technology can reduce pressures on limited staff, and increase control and choice for patients. Its use has been shown to have a positive effect on health, in enabling independence and by reducing the burden of care on informal carers (Bowes and McColgan, 2006; Gambling and Long, 2006). Furthermore, it can have a positive influence on the relationships between the patient and professionals, and/or the patient and his/her family and carers (Liddell et al, 2008).

## Telecare

The use of adaptions and equipment are an effective way of minimizing identified risk factors and enabling people to cope with the activities of daily living for longer. Simple additions, such as activity monitoring and alarm systems, can be used effectively to enable people to remain at home for much longer, when they may otherwise have required intensive support or been admitted to a long-term care facility (Liddell et al, 2008). Consider, for example, the elderly client who has short-term memory problems, who has become forgetful and turns on a gas appliance for cooking but fails to ignite it. There is a clear risk in this scenario of injury or loss of life from a gas explosion. Conventional solutions would have been to disconnect the cooker, subsequent provision of meals on wheels/microwave meals, and the initiation of a social care package. By using a gas detector which includes a shut-off valve linked to a call centre, not only is patient safety maintained, but their personal choice and independence are also maintained, as well as the potential cost benefits of not needing to provide additional social care resources. Much of the equipment provided and the assessment of need and decisions to use this come under the umbrella of social interventions, and as such are not necessarily seen as the remit of health professionals. However, it is important to remember that holistic care involves enabling the individual to maintain independence with an acceptable quality of life, and that supporting daily activities of living is an integral part of the overall solution to independent living and managing long-term conditions. Nurses, therefore, should be aware of the range, scope and availability of telecare options.

## Telehealth

The use of telehealth may be viewed as having more obvious links to health professionals in the management of long-term conditions. It involves the provision of user-friendly computerized equipment to patients in their own homes, allowing them to monitor vital signs, which can then be directly relayed through the computer/phone line to a central secure database. In addition, systems can also be used to programme reminders for patients to take their medication. There are a wide variety of monitors available which can be customized for the individual, programmed in their preferred language, and tailored to fit with their lifestyle and personal choices. These systems are clearly beneficial in facilitating the monitoring of patients across wide geographical areas and can be particularly useful for isolated communities and rural environments (Finch et al, 2008; Liddell et al, 2008). Their use in the short term can facilitate early discharge from hospital and allow for ongoing monitoring, while stabilizing the patient. In the long term, they can be useful in risk management and guide decision-making for those with unstable or fragile conditions, by providing accurate information to indicate the early signs of deterioration. The ability to provide early intervention (e.g. adjustment of medication) can prevent admission or readmission to secondary care, which can be a feature of many long-term conditions (Bayer et al, 2005). Cost benefits can also be seen for professionals in the reduced necessity for home visits and outpatient clinic reviews, and for patients in time and transport costs (Clemensen et al, 2008; Finch et al, 2008).

Evidence shows that from the patient perspective there are many positive benefits in using telehealth systems. Patients indicated that they feel more in control of their condition and empowered (Finch et al, 2008; Horton, 2008), and that this has enhanced their quality of life (Bowes and McColgan, 2006). By being involved in taking and viewing their own vital signs, patients often develop an increased awareness and understanding of their condition and as a consequence, may be better able to manage it (Finch et al, 2008; Gambling and Long, 2006). Horton (2008) notes that patients also value having a direct link at the end of a phone line and rapid access to a professional when required, which can sustain feelings that support is there when it is needed and not necessarily reliant on when the nurse arrives. Positive benefits are also evident for carers and relatives. The reassurance that their loved ones are being carefully monitored and have rapid access to support when needed can give them the confidence to go out or take a much needed break or holiday (Bowes and McColgan, 2006).

## Limitations of technology

It is, however, important that we recognize that the provision of telecare and telehealth technology may have its limitations. There are a wide variety of telehealth systems available, some fully computerized, some hard-wired, and other less invasive wireless systems. Equipment requires installation, maintenance and often requires broadband access to function. It is clear this may lead to inequities in who is able to access such systems, and therefore who is allocated these resources. However, the *Digital Britain* report (Department for Culture, Media and Sport and Department for Business, Innovation and Skills, 2009) highlights the Government's commitment to improving availability and affordability of technology; a key target of which is ensuring that everyone in the UK will be able to access broadband technology by 2012.

Effective implementation is also dependent on an ability to use the equipment and there may be difficulties, for example, for those with poor dexterity or vision (Liddell et al, 2008). Patients will require initial support and education in learning how to use each system and to develop their confidence in the safety and security of the technology. Horton (2008) noted that a barrier to effective implementation of telehealth can be the reluctance of nursing staff to embrace the technology if they lack confidence in operating the equipment correctly. Consequently, nurses monitoring these patients need the knowledge of how each system works and the confidence to use it to effectively support the patient.

Issues of patient confidentiality and security of data exchange may also be an issue of concern. Although the advantage of electronic health records, the ability to text reminders for appointments or medicines, and monitoring and relaying vital signs can have a positive impact on improving clinical outcomes, it is important to acknowledge that this may create greater risks in protecting and ensuring patient confidentiality. The risks may increase as information is more widely shared. Antai-Otong

(2007) cautions that this may lead to information not necessarily being used for the purpose for which it was intended. Effective use of the technology and access to information should be based on public and professional trust in the systems underpinned by robust policies guiding its use.

Assistive technology is championed as cost-effective; however, its success may inadvertently generate increased costs by creating new demands and increasing patient expectations on the provision and level of interventions provided (Liddell et al, 2008). There may be difficulties when withdrawing equipment from patients targeted for short-term use, who have come to rely on the technology and are subsequently reluctant to relinquish this. Liddell et al (2008) also caution that the overuse of home monitoring and testing may highlight unmet needs or lead the worried well to seek advice, further increasing the burden on already over-stretched health services.

In an increasingly technologically-driven society, face-to-face information is being replaced with electronic means. While it is easy to see that methods of communication using integrated computer technology and the remote monitoring of lifestyle allow professionals to reach more patients, there is a concern that in enabling individuals to remain in their own home by the use of such technology, those who live alone may become increasingly isolated and have little or no face-to-face human contact. We need to be careful that technology is used to enable rather than to control health care. It is important to recognize that the use of electronic technology may impact on the quality of the nurse–patient relationship (Antai-Otong, 2007), which can result in depersonalization and professional distancing (Finch et al, 2008). Although we may have facilitated the ease and speed in which information can be shared, this may lessen true communication between individuals (Antai-Otong, 2007). Professionals may perceive technological methods of communicating as less effective and less satisfying than face-to-face contact (Mair et al, 2008). Accurate diagnosis and observation often relies on verbal and non-verbal clues not necessarily conveyed via electronic means (Antai-Otong, 2007). An ability to communicate effectively and develop a good rapport with the patient is essential in effective care delivery, building trust and confidence when dealing with long-term conditions. Caring and empathy are fundamental to nursing practice, and it is difficult to convey these elements through electronic means. The use of the technology should enhance the quality of care for an individual, not replace it. Despite its advantages, technology should not entirely replace meaningful face-to-face care. The challenge for the health professional is to effectively balance the link between these differing methods of communication.

## Case study 1

*Mary is 78 years old and has lived in a small cottage in a rural village all her life. Her family lives some distance away, but try to visit at least twice a week. Recently, they have noticed that she has become very forgetful. She was hospitalized needing overnight stays on two occasions in the last year following falls. She has been seen by her GP and he has suggested that she may have the early signs of dementia. She is fiercely independent and likes to do her own cooking and shopping. Lately, however, her daughter has noticed that the food in her fridge is often not eaten. Mary relies on her neighbours who have been very supportive and often accompany her to the local store. There have been several occasions when Mary has been found wandering to the local store in the early evenings after closing time.*

## Case study 2

*Peter is 55 years old and has chronic obstructive pulmonary disease (COPD). He is divorced and now lives alone. He has two adult children who he sees infrequently, as they live in another area of the country. He lives in a ground floor local authority bungalow on an inner-city housing estate. Peter is on continuous oxygen therapy and is able to mobilize very short distances around the bungalow, but rarely leaves his home. He has regular input from home care services twice daily, who assist him in meeting his hygiene needs. He is under the care of the local community matron who monitors his condition. He has been admitted to hospital three times this year with an exacerbation of his COPD. Peter is lonely and has little contact with outside individuals, other than health and social care professionals. He often panics when he is unable to breathe and rings for an ambulance. He is currently an inpatient and is ready for discharge home.*

## Reflection

- Look at the two case studies
- What type of assistive technology might be appropriate to support these individuals to remain at home?
- What benefits might this have for the patient, the professionals, carers and relatives?
- Consider some of the patients you have met
- Could their quality of life have been improved through the use of assistive technology?

# Pathway of care

The choice and provision of technology is often quite straightforward; however, ensuring that there are effective support networks to underpin its organization, support and management within the complexities of health and social care provision is more challenging. As the use of technology becomes more commonplace in supporting and delivering effective care to individuals with long-term conditions, it may be useful to consider how a pathway approach can support its use. The provision of assistive technology requires an approach that demonstrates a coordinated pathway of care, which places the needs of the individual centrally. This process should be initiated by an appropriate assessment of need and selection of the most appropriate equipment. It requires assessment of the home environment, provision of equipment and education in its use, which should be supported by ongoing management, monitoring and review of its efficacy by knowledgeable professionals (*Table 16.2*).

---

**Table 16.2 Pathway to support use of technology**

**Assessment of need**
- Single Assessment Process/Common Assessment Framework

**Identification of care**
- Individualized care plan

**Choice of technology**
- Policies consent/confidentiality
- Identify appropriate response protocol

**Assessment of home environment**
- Home survey

**Provision of equipment**
- Installation and maintenance

**Education**
- Support for user/carer

**Monitoring and ongoing support**
- Contacts and level of input
- Professional responsibilities
- Crisis response

**Review**
- Reevaluation of need and efficacy

---

Initiatives such as the Single Assessment Process or Common Assessment Framework (DH, 2001; NHS Modernisation Agency, 2005; DH, 2009b) and individualized care planning can ensure that comprehensive assessment is undertaken. Assessment of need in complex cases may need to be jointly undertaken with both health and social care involvement. Effective communication between patient, carers and all professionals involved is essential in ensuring holistic quality care is provided. Collaboration between agencies can be beneficial in delivering coordinated and seamless care. A commitment towards partnership working between all agencies involved in health and social care can be viewed as fundamental to the effective use of assistive technologies in the management of long-term conditions.

## Conclusion

This chapter has examined how the use of assistive technology can support healthcare provision. It is evident that there is a wide range of equipment, systems and technology that can be used. It is clear that technology will play an increasing role in managing health care in the future, and there are significant benefits in using this to support independent living for individuals with ongoing health and social care needs. The use of assistive technology recognizes the rights of the individual to maintain control over his/her life and live with dignity (DH, 2005). However, it is important to remember that assistive technology is only one component of care. An individualized approach that coordinates the use of technology with more traditional methods is likely to be the best way to successfully integrate its use in the provision of health care in the future.

Antai-Otong D (2007) *Nurse-client communication: a life span approach.* Jones and Bartlett Publishers, Massachusetts

Barlow J, Singh D, Bayer S, Curry R (2007) A systematic review of the benefits of home telecare for frail elderly people and those with long-term conditions. *J Telemed Telecare* **13**(4): 172–9

Bayer S, Barlow J, Curry R (2005) *Assessing the Impact of a Care Innovation Tanaka Business School Discussion Papers TBS/DP05/38.* Tanaka Business School, London

Bowes A, McColgan G (2006) *Smart Technology and Community Care for Older People: Innovation in West Lothian.* Age Concern Scotland, Edinburgh

Clemensen J, Larsen SB, Kirkevold M, Ejskjaer N (2008) Treatment of Diabetic Foot Ulcers in the Home: Video Consultation as an Alternative to Outpatient Hospital Care.

http://tinyurl.com/yk8nbsy (accessed 1 December 2009)

Department for Culture Media and Sport (DCMS) and Department for Business Innovation and Skills (DBIS) (2009) Digital Britain: The Final Report. http://tinyurl.com/mg3o6b (accessed 1 December 2009)

DH (2001) *National Service Framework for older people*. DH, London. ref: 2001

DH (2005) *Building telecare in England*. DH, London. ref: 5217

DH (2006) Our health, our care, our say. http://tinyurl.com/yvkmdx (accessed 1 December 2009)

DH (2008a) *Raising the Profile of Long Term Conditions Care: A Compendium of Information*. DH, London. ref: 8734

DH (2008b) *High quality care for all: NHS Next Stage Review final report*. DH, London. ref: 10106

DH (2009a) Your health, your way—a guide to long term conditions and self care. http://tinyurl.com/mfua5j (accessed 1 December 2009)

DH (2009b) *Common Assessment Framework for Adults. a consultation on proposals to improve information sharing around multi-disciplinary assessment and care planning*. DH, London. ref: 11096

DH Care Networks (2009) About Telecare. http://tinyurl.com/yhwbss7 (accessed 1 December 2009)

Finch T, Mort M, Mair F, May C (2008) Future patients? Telehealthcare, roles and responsibilities. *Health Soc Care Community* **16**(1): 86–95

Gambling T, Long A (2006) Exploring patient perceptions of movement through the stages of change model within a diabetes tele-care intervention. http://tinyurl.com/ygssrxo (accessed 1 December 2009)

Horton K (2008) The use of telecare for people with chronic obstructive pulmonary disease. implications for management. *J Nurs Manag* **16**(2): 173–80

Joint Improvement Team (2008) *Telecare in Scotland Benchmarking the Present Embracing the Future*. Joint Improvement Team, Edinburgh

Liddell A, Adshead S, Burgess E (2008) *Technology in the NHS*. The King's Fund, London

Mair FS, Hiscock J, Beaton SC (2008) Understanding factors that inhibit or promote the utilization of telecare in chronic lung disease. *Chronic Ill* **4**(2): 110–7

NHS Modernisation Agency (2005) Good care planning for people with long-term conditions. http://tinyurl.com/ykdtsy8 (accessed 1 December 2009)

Skills for Health (2008) Common core principles to support self care: a guide to support implementation. http://tinyurl.com/l56g65 (accessed 1 December 2009)

WSD Action Network (2009) www.wsdactionnetwork.org.uk (accessed 1 December 2009)

# Index